Dental Drug Booklet

Handbook of Commonly Used Dental Medications

2021-2022

Peter L. Jacobsen, PhD, DDS

Diplomate, American Board of Oral Medicine
Adjunct Professor, Dept. of Dental Practice and Community Service

University of the Pacific
Arthur A. Dugoni School of Dentistry
San Francisco, CA
pgjacobs@pacbell.net
www.peterjacobsen.com

To place an order, call 1-855-633-0577
or visit https://store.wolterskluwercdi.com/CDI

NOTICE

This data is intended to serve the user as a handy reference and not as a complete drug information resource. The nature of drug information is that it is constantly evolving because of ongoing research and clinical experience and is often subject to interpretation. UpToDate, Inc. ("UpToDate") publishes summary drug information in this reference resource for use by healthcare professionals in the course of their professional practice. The content in this resource is intended only to supplement – not substitute for or replace – the knowledge and judgment of physicians, nurses, pharmacists and other healthcare professionals regarding drug therapy and patient-specific health conditions. The content is published based upon publicly available sources generally viewed as reliable in the healthcare community, including specifically pharmaceutical manufacturer labeling, information published by regulatory agencies and primary medical literature. UpToDate does not engage in any independent review, testing or study of any medication, medical device, condition, illness, injury, test, procedure, treatment, or therapy in connection with the publication of the content. The content is not intended to explicitly or implicitly endorse any particular medication as safe or effective for treating any particular patient or health condition.

Certain of UpToDate's authors, editors, reviewers, and contributors have written portions of this book in their individual capacities. The inclusion of content is not intended to indicate that it has been reviewed or endorsed by any federal or state agency, pharmaceutical company, or regulatory body. UpToDate assumes no responsibility or liability for errors or omissions of any kind in the content. UpToDate expressly disclaims any liability for any loss or damage claimed to have resulted from the use of the content. Users of the content shall hold UpToDate harmless from any such claims and shall indemnify UpToDate for any expenses incurred if such claims are made. In no event shall UpToDate nor any of its authors, editors, reviewers, contributors or publishers be liable to any user or any third-party, including specifically any customer or patient of a user, for direct, special, indirect, incidental, or consequential damages. UpToDate disclaims all warranties of any kind or nature, whether expressed or implied, including any warranty as to the quality, accuracy, comprehensiveness, currency, suitability, availability, compatibility, merchantability, and fitness for a particular purpose of the content.

If you have any suggestions or questions regarding any information presented in this data, please contact our drug information pharmacists at (855) 633-0577. Book revisions are available at our website at http://www.wolterskluwercdi.com/clinical-notices/revisions/.

© 2021 UpToDate, Inc. and its affiliates and/or licensors. All rights reserved

Printed in the United States. No part of this publication may be reproduced, stored in a retrieval system, used as a source of information for transcription into any hospital or other information system, electronic health or medical record, or transmitted in any form or by any means, electronic, mechanical, photocopying, recording or otherwise, without the prior written permission of UpToDate, Inc. Should you or your institution have a need for this information in a format we protect, we have solutions for you. Please contact our office at the number above.

ISBN: 978-1-59195-386-9

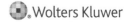

CONTENTS

SECTION I
- Prescription Writing 11
- Prescription Requirements 12
- Common Abbreviations 12
- Useful Internet Websites 13

SECTION II
- 1) Anxiety Control / Anxiolysis 17
- 2) Acute Pain 21
- 3) Infection (Bacterial) 33
- 4) Infection (Fungal) 41
- 5) Infection (Viral) 47
- 6) Oral Soft Tissue Problems 53
  - Aphthous Ulcers (Canker Sores) 54
  - ANUG or NUG 56
  - Allergy 57
  - Autoimmune Disease 58
  - Aphthous (Cauterizer) 60
  - Angular Cheilitis 60
  - Magic Mouthwash 61
- 7) Miscellaneous 63
  - Dentin Hypersensitivity 64
  - Anticaries Agents 65
  - Antiplaque and Antigingivitis Agents 71
  - Halitosis / Oral Malodor 73
  - Probiotics, Prebiotics and Oral Health 75
  - HIV-Associated Periodontal Disease 77
  - Muscle Relaxants 78
  - Periodontal Disease 79
  - Salivary Problems 80
  - Sinus Infection Treatment 83
  - Dry Socket 84
  - Pediatric Oral Dosages 85
- 8) Managing Medically Complex Patients 89
  - Prophylactic Antibiotic Coverage 90
    - Cardiac 91
  - Orthopaedic Implants 96
  - Antiresorptive Agent-Induced (Bisphosphonate) Osteonecrosis of the Jaw (ARONJ) 101
  - Pregnant and Breastfeeding Patients 103
- 9) Tobacco Cessation 107

SUBJECT INDEX

Acute Necrotizing Ulcerating Gingivitis (ANUG)	56
Allergy	57
Angular Cheilitis	60
Antiplaque and Antigingivitis Agents	71
Antiresorptive Agent-Induced (Bisphosphonate) Osteonecrosis of the Jaw	101
Anxiety Control / Anxiolysis	17
Aphthous (Cauterizer)	60
Aphthous Ulcers (Canker Sores)	54
Autoimmune Diseases (Lichen Planus, Pemphigoid, Pemphigus)	58
Bacterial Endocarditis	91
Bacterial Infections	33
Cardiac	91
Caries (Dental Decay)	65
Dentin Hypersensitivity	64
Dry Socket (Acute / Alveolar Osteitis)	84
Fungal Infections	41
Gingivitis	71
Halitosis / Oral Malodor	73
Herpes Simplex	48
HIV-Associated Periodontal Disease	77
Magic Mouthwash	61
Muscle Relaxants	78
Necrotizing Ulcerating Gingivitis (NUG)	56
Necrotizing Ulcerating Periodontitis	77
Orthopaedic Implants	96
Pain Management	22
Pediatric Oral Dosages	85
Periodontal Disease	79
Plaque	71
Pregnancy and Breastfeeding	103
Prescription Writing	11
Probiotics, Prebiotics, and Oral Health	75
Prophylactic Antibiotic Coverage	90
Saliva Blockers	82

SUBJECT INDEX

Saliva Stimulants	80
Sialorrhea	82
Sinus Infections	83
Tobacco Cessation	107
Viral Infections	47
Xerostomia	80

DRUG INDEX

Abreva	51
Acetaminophen	22, 23, 25, 86
Acetaminophen and Codeine	27, 86
Acetaminophen and Tramadol	28
Acyclovir	49, 50, 86
Advil	24
Aleve	25
Alvogyl	84
Ambien	19
Amoxicillin	38, 83, 86, 92, 99
Amoxicillin and Clavulanate	38, 83
Ampicillin	94, 99
Apo-Acetaminophen (Canada)	22, 23, 25, 86
APO-Amoxi-Clav (Canada)	38, 83
APO-Cephalex (Canada)	38, 86, 92, 99
APO-Clarithromycin (Canada)	93
APO-Clindamycin (Canada)	38, 86, 93
APO-Pen VK (Canada)	39
APO-PredniSONE (Canada)	59
Arnica Montana 30X	31
Aspirin	24
Ativan	18
Augmentin	38, 83
Azithromycin	39, 86, 93, 99, 100
Benzalkonium Chloride and Benzocaine	51
Betadine solution	56
Biotene Dry Mouth Oral Balance gel	81
Biotene Dry Mouth toothpaste	81
Bupropion	109
Cefazolin	94, 95
Ceftriaxone	94, 95, 99, 100
CeleBREX	26
Celecoxib	26
Cephalexin	38, 86, 92, 99
Cetirizine	57

DRUG INDEX

Cevimeline	80
Chantix	109
Chlorhexidine Gluconate	72, 102
Chlorhexidine-Thymol varnish	66
Clarithromycin	93
Claritin	83
Cleocin	38, 86, 93
Clindamycin	38, 86, 93
Clobetasol ointment	58
Clonazepam	78
Clotrimazole	43, 86
Colgate Total	72
Crest ProHealth	64, 72
Curcumin	31
Cyclobenzaprine	78
Dalacin C (Canada)	38, 86, 93
Debacterol	60
Denavir cream	50
Dexamethasone elixir	59
Dexasone [DSC] (Canada)	59
Diazepam	18, 87
Diflucan	45, 87
Dilaudid	29
Docosanol	51
Doxycycline	79
Entrophen (Canada)	24
Evoxac	80
Flagyl	39
Flexeril [DSC]	78
Fluconazole	45, 87
Fluocinonide ointment	58
Fluoride	68, 69, 70
Fluoride varnish	69
Halcion	18
Hydrocodone and Acetaminophen	29

DRUG INDEX

Hydrocodone and Ibuprofen	28
Hydromorphone	29
Hydroxyzine	19, 87
Ibuprofen	23, 24, 26, 87
Keflex	38, 86, 92, 99
Lidex ointment [DSC]	58
Lidocaine	49
Listerine	72
LivFresh Dental Gel	72
Loratadine	83
Lorazepam	18
Magic Mouthwash	61
Medrol	32
Methylprednisolone	32
Metronidazole	39, 87
Moi-Stir	81
Motrin	24
Mouth Kote	81
Mycelex troche [DSC]	43
Mycolog-II cream [DSC]	42, 60
Naproxen	25, 87
Neutral Sodium Fluoride gel/toothpaste	69
Novamoxin (Canada)	38, 83, 86, 92, 99
NOVO-Pen VK [DSC] (Canada)	39
Nystatin and Triamcinolone cream	42, 60
Nystatin ointment, cream, or powder	44
Nystatin oral suspension	44
Nystatin tablet	43
Orajel Touchfree Coldsore Treatment	51
Oxycodone and Acetaminophen	30
Oxycodone and Aspirin	30
Oxymetazoline	83
Penciclovir	50
Penicillin V Potassium	39
Percocet	30

DRUG INDEX

Peridex	72
PerioGard	72
Periostat (Canada)	79
Pilocarpine Hydrochloride	80
Potassium Nitrate	64
Povidone-Iodine	56
Prednisone	59
PreviDent Varnish	69
Propantheline	82
Salagen	80
Saliva Blockers	82
Saliva Stimulants	80
Saliva Substitutes	81
Silver Diamine Fluoride	67
Sodium Fluoride	68, 69
Stannous Fluoride	70
Sulfonated Phenolics and Sulfuric Acid	60
Temovate ointment	58
Tempra (Canada)	22, 23, 25, 86
TEVA-Nystatin (Canada)	43
TEVA-Oxycodan (Canada)	30
Triamcinolone paste	58
Triazolam	18
Tylenol	25
Tylenol #2, #3, #4	27
Tylenol with Codeine #3	27
Ultracet	28
Valacyclovir	48, 50
Valium	18, 87
Valtrex	50
Varenicline	109
Verdrocet	29
Vicodin [DSC]	29
Viroxyn	51
Vistaril	19, 07

DRUG INDEX

Wellbutrin SR	109
Xodol	29
Xylitol	66
Xylocaine 2% Viscous	48, 49
Zithromax (Tri-Pak, Z-Pak)	39
Zolpidem	19
Zovirax	48, 50
Zyban [DSC]	109
ZyrTEC	57

SECTION I

PRESCRIPTION WRITING

Doctor's Name

Address

Phone Number

Patient's Name   Date

Patient's Address   Age

Rx   Drug Name   Dosage/Size

Disp   Number of tablets, capsules, ounces to be dispensed. (Roman numerals may be added as precaution for commonly abused drugs).

            The amount of drug prescribed is the responsibility of the prescribing clinician and is based on their estimate of individual patient need – see **NOTE** on page 21.

Sig   Directions on how the drug is to be taken.

Doctor's Signature

State License Number

DEA Number   (if required)

Generic   (This note, if appropriate, added to the prescription, allows the pharmacist to fill with the least expensive generic drug available.)

NOTE: The prescriptions in this booklet are intended for the adult population. Pediatric dosage is indicated when appropriate with a note to see the Pediatric Oral Dosage table on pages 85 to 87.

PRESCRIPTION REQUIREMENTS

1) Date
2) Full name, address, and date of birth of patient (some states also require patient's weight)
3) Name and address of prescriber
4) Signature of prescriber

If class II, III, IV drug, a Drug Enforcement Agency (DEA) number is necessary.

If a DEA class II-V drug, in the state of California and several other states, a special tamper-proof prescription form printed only by state-approved printers is required. Check with your state dental society for details and contact information for authorized printers. **Note:** These prescription forms are required for all class II-IV drugs, but can also be used for all prescriptions.

COMMON ABBREVIATIONS

i, ii, iii	one, two, three
q	every (as in "every" 6 hours)
d	day
h	hour
prn	as needed
stat	at once, immediately
bid	twice daily
tid	three times a day
qid	four times a day

Example: tid = 3 times a day
q8h = every 8 hours

**ABBREVIATIONS CAN BE ERROR-PRONE,
IF IN DOUBT, WRITE IT OUT!**

For more information about avoiding dangerous, error-prone abbreviations, see http://www.ismp.org/tools/errorproneabbreviations.pdf

USEFUL INTERNET WEBSITES

American Association of Orthopedic Surgeons, American Dental Association,
   March 2013, Prevention of Orthopaedic Implant Infection in Patients Undergoing Dental
      Procedures
      https://www.ada.org/en/member-center/oral-health-topics/antibiotic-prophylaxis
      http://www.orthoguidelines.org/go/auc/default.cfm?auc_id=224995&actionxm=Terms
      http://www.ada.org/en/publications/ada-news/viewpoint/my-view/2013/january/my-view
         (*interesting and worthwhile discussion on the development of the guidelines*)

American Dental Association, Antibiotic Prophylaxis guidelines in dentistry
      http://www.ada.org/en/member-center/oral-health-topics/antibiotic-prophylaxis
      http://www.ada.org/~/media/ada/advocacy/files/anesthesia_use_guidelines.pdf?la=en
      https://www.ahajournals.org/doi/10.1161/CIR.0000000000000969

American Heart Association Guidelines for the Prevention of Infective Endocarditis, April 2007
      https://www.ahajournals.org/doi/10.1161/circulationaha.106.183095

Dental Management Protocols for Medically Complex Patients and HIV-Infected Patients;
   as well as a health history translated into 40 languages and a health history interview sheet.
      http://www.dental.pacific.edu/departments-and-groups/professional-services-and-
         resources/dental-practice-documents

National Institute of Dental and Craniofacial Research
   Information on a wide range of dental problems and their management
      https://www.nidcr.nih.gov/health-info

   Organ Transplant Patient Management Suggestions
      https://www.in.gov/isdh/files/OrganTransplantProf.pdf

Website to purchase the Little Dental Drug Booklet
      https://store.wolterskluwercdi.com/CDI

Note: Links to specific sites and/or documents can change unpredictably so please accept my apologies if the link does not work. You can email me with any questions (pgjacobs@pacbell.net).

SECTION II

Situations and the Appropriate Medications to Be Used

1) ANXIETY CONTROL/ ANXIOLYSIS

Diazepam (Valium)
Hydroxyzine (Vistaril)
Lorazepam (Ativan)
Triazolam (Halcion)
Zolpidem (Ambien)

NOTE:

Anxiolysis, the decrease of anxiety in a fully alert and responsive patient, requires no permit. The following medications are for anxiolysis.

Sedation, the mental and physiological slowing of the patient with medication may require a special permit in some states depending on the age of the patient and the level of sedation. If you intend to use medication to sedate a patient, you should acquire training and certification in such procedures.

In California, and possibly other states (check your state law), Oral sedation means anything given by mouth that will sedate or relax the patient. This would include sedative / hypnotics (benzodiazepines, barbiturates), antihistamines, opioids, and chloral hydrate.

MEDICATIONS: ANXIETY CONTROL/ANXIOLYSIS

Rx	**Diazepam*** (Valium) **5 mg**
Disp	4 tablets
Sig	Take 1 tablet in evening before going to bed and 1 tablet 1 hour before your appointment

CAUTION: Patient should not drive themselves to or from the appointment. Do not prescribe to pregnant women. Dose adjustment may be appropriate in the elderly or medically complex patients.

NOTE: Half-life: 44 to 100 hours

Rx	**Lorazepam** (Ativan) **1 mg**
Disp	2 tablets
Sig	Take 1 tablet in evening before going to bed and 1 tablet 1 hour before your appointment

CAUTION: As for Valium

NOTE: Half-life: ~12 hours

Rx	**Triazolam** (Halcion) **0.25 mg**
Disp	4 tablets
Sig	Take 1 tablet in evening before going to bed and 1 tablet 1 hour before your appointment

CAUTION: As for Valium

NOTE: Half-life: 1.5 to 5.5 hours

MEDICATIONS: ANXIETY CONTROL/ANXIOLYSIS

Rx **Hydroxyzine* (Vistaril) 25 mg**

Disp 8 capsules

Sig Take 2 capsules in evening before going to bed and 2 capsules 1 hour before your appointment

CAUTION: Patient should not drive themselves to or from the appointment.

NOTE: Half-life: ~20 hours

Rx **Zolpidem (Ambien) 5 mg**

Disp 2 tablets

Sig Take 1 tablet 30 minutes before appointment

CAUTION: Patient should not drive themselves to or from the appointment.

NOTE: Some patients may require a 10 mg dose

No drug is completely safe during pregnancy and zolpidem does cross the placental barrier which can adversely affect/sedate the unborn child.

Ambien is rated safer for pregnant patients than the benzodiazepines. With zolpidem's short half-life (~3 hours), experience in pregnant patients, and single use for a dental procedure, it makes a reasonable choice when indicated.

*For pediatric dosage, see pages 85 to 87.

2) ACUTE PAIN

Mild to Moderate
- Acetaminophen
- Aspirin
- Celecoxib (CeleBREX)
- Ibuprofen
- Naproxen (Aleve)

Moderate to Severe
- Acetaminophen and Codeine
- Acetaminophen and Tramadol (Ultracet)
- Hydrocodone and Acetaminophen
- Hydrocodone and Ibuprofen

Severe
- Hydromorphone (Dilaudid)
- Oxycodone and Acetaminophen (Percocet)
- Oxycodone and Aspirin

All prescription opioid pain medications can be filled generically.

NOTE: The number of tablets suggested in the "Disp" section of the prescriptions in this booklet are just that, *suggestions* for the **average patient**. The practitioner should prescribe as many tablets as needed based on the amount and duration of pain or problems expected by each individual patient. Keep in mind that prescribing too many tablets, especially opioids, can have detrimental effects, so proper judgment is important. The risk of too few tablets is less than the risk of too many, especially when prescribing opioids for severe pain. If the pain or problem is persisting longer than expected, having the patient contact you is better than them taking a medication that is not working for too long a time.

NOTE: <u>Chronic Head and Neck Pain</u> is a complex diagnostic and therapeutic problem. If you do not have special training in this area, refer patient to a dentist or physician who does.

PAIN MANAGEMENT IN DENTISTRY

All states require dentists to possess a DEA registration and many states also have a drug tracking system they are encouraged to utilize. Dentists should check their state's requirements.

Dentists are advised to check the controlled substance record/drug tracking system for all new patient opioid prescriptions and any time a patient appears to require, or they request, more than 3 days of opioid medication.

Because of a national epidemic of opioid abuse, the Center for Disease Control has provided guidelines (March 2016) for primarily chronic opioid prescribing/utilization. These recommendations also include advice for acute opioid use, which is the most common need in dental practice. They suggest that opioid use be limited to 3 days and that the maximum prescribed amount should not exceed 7 days. Leftover drugs from dental prescriptions have been implicated as an initial source of opioids in a large number of what is now called opioid use disorder, previously called narcotic addiction.

ACETAMINOPHEN WARNING:

1. Warn patient not to combine acetaminophen-containing opioid combinations with over-the-counter acetaminophen or other acetaminophen-containing products such as NyQuil and some Theraflu products.
2. Do not exceed a maximum single dose of 650 mg of acetaminophen (in opioid combination) or a maximum daily dose of 4 g. If patient has liver disease, consult with MD and consider lower daily maximum in elderly patients, patients with history of alcohol use, and those with impaired liver function (https://www.ncbi.nlm.nih.gov/pubmed/?term=19573219).

PAIN MANAGEMENT DECISION MAKING

Most pain in dentistry is in the "mild to moderate" range. The nonsteroidal anti-inflammatory drugs, combined with acetaminophen, are a very powerful pain control combination and should be used first for dental pain or in anticipation of dental pain secondary to a dental procedure.

ASPIRIN TOLERANT:

Ibuprofen
200 to 600 mg 4 times a day
(breakfast, lunch, dinner, and before bed)

Start medication at time of the procedure and use for next several days to prevent pain from starting (preemptive analgesia). Ibuprofen is a very effective pain medication, especially for inflammatory / dental pain.

If pain is not controlled, then add on **acetaminophen** 500 mg to the ibuprofen dose.

If pain is severe, then drop the acetaminophen and add on **hydrocodone and acetaminophen** combination product to the ibuprofen (ie, 2 tablets [hydrocodone 5 mg and acetaminophen 300 mg/tablet]).

If pain is very severe (ie, dry socket or equivalent), consider **oxycodone and acetaminophen** (ie, 1 to 2 Percocet [oxycodone 5 to 10 mg and acetaminophen 325 mg/tablet]).

The above opioids should only be used for 24 to 72 hours along with the ibuprofen, then back to the less powerful drugs. **Do not exceed acetaminophen 4 g daily.**

ASPIRIN ALLERGIC / INTOLERANT:

Acetaminophen* (OTC) (see *Warning on page 22)
650 mg 4 times a day (not to exceed 4 g per 24 hours)

If pain is not controlled, stop acetaminophen and switch to: codeine and acetaminophen (**Tylenol #3**), hydrocodone and acetaminophen, or tramadol and acetaminophen (**Ultracet**).

If pain is very severe (ie, dry socket or equivalent), consider: oxycodone and acetaminophen (**Percocet**) or equivalent for 24 to 72 hours.

MEDICATIONS: PAIN (MILD-MODERATE) OTC
Available over-the-counter (OTC)
Nonsteroidal anti-inflammatory drugs (NSAIDs)

Rx	**Aspirin 325 mg (OTC)**

Disp   To be determined by practitioner

Sig   1 to 2 tablets every 4 to 6 hours (maximum adult dose: 4 g 24 hours)

> **NOTE:** See Note 2 under Ibuprofen below – it applies to all NSAIDs including aspirin.

Rx	**Ibuprofen 200 mg (OTC)**

Disp   To be determined by practitioner

Sig   1 to 3 tablets every 4 to 6 hours (prescription maximum adult dose: 3,200 mg/24 hours)

> **NOTE 1:** Ibuprofen is available over-the-counter as Motrin IB, Advil, and many other brands in 200 mg tablets.
>
> **NOTE 2:**
> a) NSAIDs should never be taken together, nor combined with aspirin. NSAIDs have anti-inflammatory effects as well as producing analgesia.
>
> b) An allergy / intolerance to aspirin constitutes a relative contraindication to all NSAIDs.
>
> c) All NSAIDs can be taken with food to minimize risk of stomach upset. Aspirin and the NSAIDs may increase post-treatment bleeding and GI bleeding.
>
> d) Risk of cardiovascular thrombotic events, including stroke and MI, as well as HTN, may increase with duration of use, especially in those with preexisting cardiovascular risk factors or disease.

MEDICATIONS: PAIN (MILD-MODERATE) OTC
Available over-the-counter (OTC)
Nonsteroidal anti-inflammatory drugs (NSAIDs)

Rx	**Naproxen** (Aleve) **(OTC)**
Disp	To be determined by practitioner
Sig	Take 2 tablets to start, then take 1 tablet every 8 to 12 hours up to 3 tablets (660 mg) per day

INGREDIENT: Naproxen sodium 220 mg/tablet

NOTE: See Note 2 under Ibuprofen on page 24 – it applies to all NSAIDs.

MEDICATIONS: PAIN (MILD-MODERATE) OTC
Available over-the-counter (OTC)
(For patients allergic to aspirin and other NSAIDs)

Rx	**Acetaminophen 325 mg (OTC)**
Disp	To be determined by practitioner
Sig	Take 500 to 650 mg every 4 to 6 hours

PRODUCTS INCLUDE: Tylenol, Mapap, and many others

NOTE:
1. Acetaminophen can be given if patient has allergy, bleeding problems, risk factors/contraindications, or stomach upset secondary to aspirin or NSAIDs.

2. Warn patient not to combine acetaminophen-containing opioid combinations such as Percocet, Vicodin, Ultracet, and Tylenol #3 with over-the-counter acetaminophen or other acetaminophen-containing products such as NyQuil and some Theraflu products.

3. Do not exceed a maximum single dose of 650 mg of acetaminophen (in opioid combination), or a maximum daily dose of 4 g.

MEDICATIONS: PAIN (MILD-MODERATE) Rx
Require Prescription (Rx)
Nonsteroidal anti-inflammatory drugs (NSAIDs)

Rx **Ibuprofen 600 mg**

Disp 28 tablets

Sig Take 1 tablet 3 times per day

> **NOTE:** For severe pain, 600 mg can be given up to 4 times per day.
>
> Maximum adult dose: 3,200 mg/24 hours
>
> The above is the prescription dose. The same dosage can be accomplished using 3 of the 200 mg over-the-counter tablets.

Rx **Celecoxib** (CeleBREX) **200 mg**

Disp 15 capsules

Sig Take 2 capsules stat, followed by an additional capsule (200 mg) as needed on day 1, then 1 capsule every 12 hours

> **NOTE:** May be beneficial in patients with history of previous peptic ulcer disease.

NOTE: See Note 2 under Ibuprofen on page 24 - it applies to all NSAIDs.

MEDICATIONS: PAIN (MODERATE-SEVERE)
All opioids are "scheduled" and require DEA license to prescribe

The following is a guideline to use when prescribing codeine with acetaminophen [300 mg/tablet] (Tylenol):

>Codeine No. 2 = Codeine 15 mg
>Codeine No. 3 = Codeine 30 mg
>Codeine No. 4 = Codeine 60 mg

Rx	**Acetaminophen* and Codeine** (Tylenol with Codeine #3)
Disp	16 tablets
Sig	Take 1 tablet every 4 to 6 hours as needed for pain
	INGREDIENTS: Acetaminophen 300 mg; Codeine 30 mg
	NOTE: Do not exceed acetaminophen 4 g/codeine 360 mg in 24 hours. For pediatric liquid preparation, see page 86 under Pediatric Oral Dosages.
	SCHEDULE III

See Acetaminophen Warning on page 22.

NOTE: The above can be filled generically.

MEDICATIONS: PAIN (MODERATE-SEVERE)
All opioids are "scheduled" and require DEA license to prescribe

Rx	**Hydrocodone and Ibuprofen**
Disp	16 tablets
Sig	Take 1 tablet every 4 to 6 hours as needed for pain

    INGREDIENTS: Hydrocodone 7.5 mg; Ibuprofen 200 mg
NOTE: Do not exceed 5 tablets in 24 hours
SCHEDULE: II

Rx	**Acetaminophen* and Tramadol** (Ultracet)
Disp	36 tablets
Sig	Take 2 tablets every 4 to 6 hours

    INGREDIENTS: Acetaminophen 325 mg; Tramadol 37.5 mg
NOTE: Do not exceed 8 tablets in 24 hours. Treatment should not exceed 5 days.
SCHEDULE: IV

***See Acetaminophen Warning** on page 22.

NOTE: All of the above can be filled generically.

MEDICATIONS: PAIN (MODERATE-SEVERE)
All opioids are "scheduled" and require DEA license to prescribe

Rx	**Hydrocodone and Acetaminophen***
Disp	16 tablets
Sig	Take 1 to 2 tablets 4 times/day as needed for pain
	INGREDIENTS: Hydrocodone 5 mg; Acetaminophen 300 mg
	OTHER BRAND NAMES: Verdrocet, Xodol, various generics (APAP dose varies between 300 to 325 mg)
	NOTE: Do not exceed 4 g acetaminophen/day
	SCHEDULE: II

*See **Acetaminophen Warning** on page 22.

MEDICATIONS: PAIN (SEVERE)
All opioids are "scheduled" and require DEA license to prescribe

Rx	**Hydromorphone** (Dilaudid) **2 mg**
Disp	16 tablets
Sig	Take 1 to 2 tablets every 4 to 6 hours for pain
	SCHEDULE: II

MEDICATIONS: PAIN (SEVERE)

All opioids are "scheduled" and require DEA license to prescribe

Rx	**Oxycodone and Aspirin**
Disp	16 tablets
Sig	Take 1 tablet every 6 hours for pain

    INGREDIENTS: Oxycodone 4.84 mg; Aspirin 325 mg
    NOTE: Do not exceed 12 tablets in 24 hours
    See Note 2 under Ibuprofen on page 24.
    SCHEDULE: II

Rx	**Oxycodone and Acetaminophen*** (Percocet) **5 mg**
Disp	16 tablets
Sig	Take 1 to 2 tablets every 6 hours for pain

    INGREDIENTS: Oxycodone 5 mg; Acetaminophen 325 mg
    OTHER BRAND NAMES: Nalocet, Prolate (contains acetaminophen 300 mg tablet), or generic equivalent
    NOTE: Do not exceed 4 g acetaminophen/day
    SCHEDULE: II

*See Acetaminophen Warning on page 22.

NOTE: All of the above can be filled generically.

MEDICATIONS: PAIN
(Other management modalities)

The foundation of pain management in dentistry is anti-inflammatory drugs and acetaminophen. When indicated, a short course of narcotics (2 to 3 days) can be appropriate. For a variety of reasons it may not be possible for some or any of those medications to be used by the patient, or the dentist may feel those drugs are not appropriate. In such cases, or in conjunction with the above, "natural" therapies may considered or, depending on your training, corticosteroids.

Rx	**Arnica Montana 30x (homeopathic preparation only)**
Disp	40 tablets
Sig	Dissolve 4 tablets under tongue 1 hour before appt and continue dissolving 4 tablets under tongue 4 times a day thereafter, for 3 days

Rx	**Curcumin 500 mg**
Disp	14 capsules
Sig	Take 1 capsule 2 times a day
	INGREDIENT: Curcumin (The active anti-inflammatory ingredient in Tumeric); The concentration varies, so look closely at the packaging for the Curcumin content. If available, find curcumin combined with piperine, for better curcumin absorption.

MEDICATIONS: PAIN
(Other management modalities)

Corticosteroids

These drugs are used for their anti-inflammatory effect to reduce swelling and pain, most commonly following endodontic procedures or dental extractions. There is no consensus as to their effectiveness or benefit. They also blunt the body's immune response thereby increasing the risk of infection. Based on the risk of infection and other side effects, I would **not** suggest their use unless you have specialty training and were taught the indications and, perhaps more importantly, contraindications for their use during that training.

Rx	**Methylprednisolone** (Medrol) **4 mg**
Disp	5 tablets
Sig	Take 1 tablet 1 hour before appointment and 1 tablet at breakfast and lunch for the next 2 days

3) INFECTION (Bacterial)

Amoxicillin
Amoxicillin and Clavulanate (Augmentin)
Azithromycin (Zithromax)
Cephalexin (Keflex)
Clindamycin (Cleocin)
Metronidazole (Flagyl)
Penicillin V Potassium

MANAGEMENT OF A DENTAL BACTERIAL INFECTION

1. Make the correct diagnosis:
   a. Signs and symptoms of an oral bacterial infection: Swelling, often pain and radiolucency, associated with teeth or gums.
   b. Signs and symptoms of a systemic bacterial infection; the above, plus fever, and often malaise.

2. Management of infection before antibiotics:
   a. Most direct and effective treatment; incise and drain/irrigate.
   b. Perform the endodontic procedure, extract the tooth, or debride the pocket (scrape off the barnacles), and incise and drain the pus pocket.

3. Decision to add antibiotics into the management of the infection:

   If the patient has swelling plus fever or other systemic manifestations and/or patient is immunocompromised, prescribing antibiotics in addition to removal of the nidus of infection would be prudent.

4. Prophylactic antibiotics are seldom, if ever, necessary for extraction or endodontic procedure in healthy patients not showing systemic manifestations of a bacterial infection. If you feel it is needed, then a one-time loading dose, consistent with the AHA recommendations for the heart (see page 91), is the appropriate choice to establish blood levels during the duration of the bacteremia caused by the procedure. Antibiotics for the following 2 to 5 days has not been documented as being of any additional benefit compared to risks and side effects.

Good Antibiotic Stewardship means prescribing the <u>correct antibiotic</u> at the <u>correct dose</u>, for the <u>correct amount of time</u>.

MANAGEMENT OF A DENTAL BACTERIAL INFECTION

NOTE: Due to safety concerns, clindamycin is no longer considered the drug of choice for patients allergic to the penicillins and is not the alternative choice if penicillin is ineffective in patients without penicillin allergy history.

We are lucky to have a safe and predictably effective antibiotic group, the penicillins, to manage dental infections. This is why they remain drug of choice in those without penicillin allergy. But we don't have many safe and effective options to choose from if a patient is allergic to penicillin, intolerant to penicillin, or the infection is unresponsive to penicillin. Recommendations changed in the Fall of 2019.

As you may have noted, the prophylaxis guidelines for patients with prosthetic joints, published in 2017, no longer recommended clindamycin as a drug of choice if the patient is allergic to penicillin. The American Association of Endodontics in the Fall of 2019 published an update to their very influential 2017 publication, Antibiotics in Dentistry. **The update states that clindamycin is no longer the best drug of choice for dental infections for patients allergic to penicillin and it is not the best second drug of choice if the infection does not respond to penicillin/amoxicillin. The new antibiotic recommendation for patients allergic to penicillin is azithromycin (Zithromax). The new recommendation for the second drug of choice if penicillin/amoxicillin is not effective is to add clavulanate potassium (a compound that inhibits penicillinase) to amoxicillin. This is commercially available as Augmentin, but is also generically available.**

The change is because of safety. Clindamycin is still a very effective antibiotic against organisms commonly associated with dental infections, and it is still the most effective antibiotic if an infection does not respond to penicillin/amoxicillin alone. The reason it is no longer recommended is

MANAGEMENT OF A DENTAL BACTERIAL INFECTION

because of its effect on the GI tract and its causality with *Clostridioides difficile* infection (CDI). It is no longer considered a safe drug to be used as the first drug of choice in patients with a penicillin allergy, and it is not a safe enough drug to use if penicillin or amoxicillin is not effective.

As noted, clindamycin is still a very effective drug and may be needed in some situations, such as when a penicillin allergic patient starts with azithromycin and it does not work. **Antibiotic choice, like all things in dentistry and medicine, always depends on the informed clinical judgement of the dentist/clinician. Depending on the severity of the infection, even with the risk of CDI, clindamycin may be the safest, most effective drug to stop the infection.** If that decision is made, clindamycin must be used knowing that it can cause serious side effects and even death. The decision to use it must be taken weighing the risk of the side effects against the risk of the infection progressing. **The dentist should inform the patient of their choice and why, and that if the patient gets serious stomach upset or diarrhea they should stop the medication and contact you and/or their physician.**

ANTIBIOTIC DECISION MAKING

1. Common drugs of choice for dental infections:

    Penicillin VK or **Amoxicillin**

2. If no response in 48 to 72 hours then use:

    A. Amoxicillin and Clavulanate (Augmentin)

    or **B. Cephalexin**

    or **C.** Some dentists elect to add **Metronidazole** to the **Amoxicillin**

3. If no response to choice **B** or **C** in 24 to 48 hours then use:

    Clindamycin

    (Be sure to incise and drain and/or irrigate, if appropriate)

IF PATIENT IS ALLERGIC TO PENICILLIN

1. First common drug of choice is:

    Azithromycin (Zithromax)

2. If no response in 48 to 72 hours then use:

    Clindamycin

NOTE: If no response to above protocol, refer to or consult with an oral-maxillofacial surgeon, endodontist, periodontist, or infectious disease physician.

If infection persists and patient is taking bone-antiresorptive drugs, such as bisphosphonate, then consider the possibility of antiresorptive drug-associated osteonecrosis.

See page 83 for sinus infection treatment.

MEDICATIONS: INFECTION (BACTERIAL)*

Rx	**Amoxicillin 500 mg**
Disp	30 tablets
Sig	Take 1 tablet 3 times per day

>**NOTE:** Loading dose is appropriate and is double the maintenance dose.

Rx	**Amoxicillin and Clavulanate** (Augmentin) **500/125 mg**
Disp	30 tablets
Sig	Take 1 tablet 3 times per day

>INGREDIENTS: Amoxicillin 500 mg and Clavulanate Potassium 125 mg
>
>**NOTE:** Augmentin is amoxicillin protected from penicillinase breakdown by clavulanate. Loading dose is appropriate and is double the maintenance dose.

Rx	**Cephalexin** (Keflex) **500 mg**
Disp	40 capsules
Sig	Take 1 capsule 4 times per day

Rx	**Clindamycin** (Cleocin) **300 mg**
Disp	30 capsules
Sig	Take 1 capsule 3 times per day

>**NOTE:** **Use with extreme caution as *C. difficile* infection can be severe. Reserved for serious infections where less toxic antibiotics are inadequate.**

*For pediatric dosage, see pages 85 to 87.

MEDICATIONS: INFECTION (BACTERIAL)*

Rx   **Metronidazole** (Flagyl) **500 mg**

Disp   40 tablets

Sig   Take 1 tablet 4 times per day

> **NOTE:** Warn patient to avoid alcohol ingestion while taking metronidazole as an interaction may occur.

Rx   **Penicillin V Potassium 500 mg**

Disp   40 tablets

Sig   Take 1 tablet 4 times per day

Rx   **Azithromycin** (Zithromax Tri-Pak) **500 mg**

Disp   1 pack

Sig   Take 1 tablet per day for 3 days

> **NOTE:** Also comes as Zithromax Z-Pak (250 mg tablets), 5 day dosing
>
> Azithromycin has been associated with QT-interval prolongation and heart arrhythmias, especially in patients with cardiovascular events and/or electrolyte abnormalities (do not use, or use with caution in these patients).

For pediatric dosage, see pages 85 to 87.

4) INFECTION (Fungal)

Clotrimazole (formerly Mycelex)
Fluconazole (Diflucan)
Nystatin (ointment, cream, oral suspension, powder, tablets)

ANTIFUNGAL DECISION MAKING

*COMMON DRUGS OF CHOICE FOR ORAL FUNGAL INFECTIONS**

The first common drugs of choice for local treatment of oral fungal infections are:

Clotrimazole (formerly Mycelex) **troche** or
Nystatin tablets

The common drug of choice for systematic treatment of oral fungal infections is:

Fluconazole (Diflucan)

The common drug of choice for angular cheilitis is:

Nystatin and Triamcinolone cream (formerly Mycolog-II)
(Rx on page 60)

NOTE: Chlorhexidine Gluconate oral rinse (Rx on page 72) has been shown to be of value to help control oral fungal infections especially immunosuppressed HIV-infected patients. (Symptomatic patients rinse 2 times per day; asymptomatic patients rinse 1 time per day at night.)

---

* For pediatric dosage, see pages 85 to 87.

MEDICATIONS: INFECTION (FUNGAL)

Rx	**Clotrimazole (Oral)** (formerly Mycelex) **troche 10 mg**
Disp	70 troches
Sig	Dissolve 1 troche in mouth 5 times/day until gone; leave any prosthesis out during treatment and soak prosthesis in nystatin liquid suspension overnight

> **NOTE:** The troche may contain sucrose, risk of caries with prolonged use (>3 months) especially if mouth is dry (see caries management in Anticaries Agents on pages 65 to 70).

Rx	**Nystatin tablets**
Disp	30 tablets
Sig	Dissolve 1 tablet in mouth until gone, 4 times per day

INGREDIENT: 500,000 units of nystatin per tablet

> **NOTE:** The soluble tablet is more effective than an oral suspension, but is sometimes hard to find.

MEDICATIONS: INFECTION (FUNGAL)

Rx **Nystatin oral suspension**

Disp 300 mL

Sig Use 1 teaspoonful for 2 minutes 4 times per day and expectorate

INGREDIENT: Nystatin 100,000 units/mL; vehicle contains 50% sucrose and not more than 1% alcohol.

NOTE: High risk of dental decay with prolonged use (>3 months). There may be an additional benefit in soaking any dental appliance in a small amount of the antifungal suspension overnight for 2 to 5 days.

Rx **Nystatin cream, ointment, or powder - select one**

Disp 15 g or 30 g tube

Sig Apply liberally to affected areas 2 to 3 times per day

INGREDIENTS:

Cream: 100,000 units nystatin per gram, aqueous vanishing cream base

Ointment: 100,000 units nystatin per gram, polyethylene and mineral oil gel base

Powder: 100,000 units nystatin per gram; may be sprinkled into dentures

MEDICATIONS: INFECTION (FUNGAL)

Rx	**Fluconazole** (Diflucan) **100 mg**
Disp	16 tablets
Sig	Take 2 tablets the first day and 1 tablet each day thereafter until resolved

> **NOTE:** To be used if *Candida* infection does not respond to local oral drug.

5) INFECTION (Viral)

Acyclovir (Zovirax)
Benzalkonium Chloride and Benzocaine
Docosanol (Abreva)
Lidocaine 2% Viscous
Penciclovir (Denavir)
Valacyclovir (Valtrex)

HERPES SIMPLEX MANAGEMENT

Oral herpes simplex is a viral disease. Secondary attacks occur primarily on lips, but when they occur inside the mouth, they occur as clusters of pinpoint ulcers on attached (overlying bone) mucosa. Aphthous ulcers are not herpes. Aphthous ulcers occur primarily on unattached mucosa (see pages 54 to 55).

PRIMARY ATTACK

- **Lidocaine 2% Viscous** (palliative)
- **Valacyclovir** (Valtrex) (best if started within 3 days of onset)
- Fluids and liquid food supplements

SECONDARY ATTACK

- **Valacyclovir** at first indication of attack (burning, tingling)
- May supplement with topical **Acyclovir** (Zovirax) ointment or **Penciclovir** (Denavir) and/or **Docosanol** (Abreva) as needed.
- Treatment of secondary herpes infections should begin as soon as the patient realizes an attack is starting. These listed antiviral drugs are very stable and can be kept on hand at home for years.

PROPHYLAXIS: ACUTE

- **Valacyclovir** 500 mg, 4 tablets twice daily (or 1,000 mg, 2 tablets twice daily) for 1 day (separate doses by 12 hours); therapy should be initiated at the first sign of any prodrome such as tingling, burning, or itching.

PROPHYLAXIS: CHRONIC (Suppressive Therapy)

- **Valacyclovir** and **Acyclovir (Systemic)** have both been used effectively and safely for the long-term management of HSV infection. Please consider a consultation with the patient's physician if you feel such treatment is appropriate.

MEDICATIONS: INFECTION (VIRAL)

Rx **Lidocaine 2% Viscous**

Disp 100 mL

Sig Use 15 mL to rinse around oral cavity no more than every 3 hours as needed to relieve pain then expectorate (do not exceed 8 doses/day)

Rx **Acyclovir 200 mg (Initial episode HSV infection)***

Disp 50 to 60 capsules

Sig Take 1 capsule 5 times per day for 7 to 10 days

Rx **Acyclovir 200 mg (Recurrent episode HSV infection)***

Disp 50 capsules**

Sig Take 1 capsule 5 times per day for 5 days (begin at the earliest signs of disease)

*Alternative options are available for immunocompetent patients.

**The dispensed number of capsules/tablets for recurrent herpes episodes are double the amount needed for 1 episode. The additional tablets/capsules are available to take at the first sign of a subsequent episode, which is very important for the effectiveness of the medication.

MEDICATIONS: INFECTION (VIRAL)

Rx	**Acyclovir** (Zovirax) **Ointment 5%**
Disp	15 g
Sig	Apply thin layer to lesion 5 times per day for 4 days

Rx	**Penciclovir** (Denavir) **Cream 1%**
Disp	5 g
Sig	Apply every 2 hours during waking hours for a period of 4 days

Rx	**Valacyclovir** (Valtrex) **500 mg**
Disp	16 tablets**
Sig	Take 4 tablets at first sign of attack and then take 4 tablets 12 hours later

NOTE: Not for HIV patients; may cause thrombocytopenia.

**The dispensed number of capsules/tablets for recurrent herpes episodes are double the amount needed for 1 episode. The additional tablets/capsules are available to take at the first sign of a subsequent episode, which is very important for the effectiveness of the medication.

MEDICATIONS: INFECTION (VIRAL)

Rx **Docosanol** (Abreva) **(OTC) Cream 10%**

Disp 2 g

Sig   Apply to lesion 5 times per day; start at first sign of cold sore or fever blister and continue until healed.

Rx **Benzalkonium Chloride and Benzocaine**

Disp 2 tubes

Sig   Saturate the applicator with solution and rub ulcer/starting herpes lesion with applicator until it becomes numb. Single treatment is usually enought for most sores, but may repeat up to 3 times daily.

INGREDIENTS: Benzalkonium Chloride 0.13% and Benzocaine 7.5%

NOTE: Available as multiple brands: Viroxyn, Orajel Touchfree Coldsore Treatment

6) ORAL SOFT TISSUE PROBLEMS

Aphthous Ulcers	**Dexamethasone** elixir **Fluocinonide** ointment (formerly Lidex) **Clobetasol** ointment (Temovate) **Triamcinolone** paste
Necrotizing Ulcerating Gingivitis	**Povidone-Iodine** (Betadine)
Allergy	**Cetirizine (Systemic)** (ZyrTEC)
Oral Autoimmune Disease (Lichen Planus, Pemphigoid, Pemphigus)	**Dexamethasone** elixir **Fluocinonide** ointment (formerly Lidex) **Prednisone** **Clobetasol** ointment (Temovate) **Triamcinolone** paste
Aphthous (Cauterizer)	**Sulfonated Phenolics and Sulfuric Acid** (Debacterol)
Angular Cheilitis	**Nystatin and Triamcinolone** cream (formerly Mycolog-II)
Magic Mouthwash	

APHTHOUS ULCERS (CANKER SORES) MANAGEMENT

Aphthous is considered an autoimmune disease with poorly understood triggering causes. The lesions occur exclusively on <u>unattached</u> (cheek, floor of mouth, etc) mucosa (as opposed to secondary herpes simplex, which intraorally, occurs only on <u>attached</u> mucosa).

Treatment for canker sores is divided into 3 sections:
1. Prevention
2. Pain relief
3. Pharmacological treatment

PREVENTION

Avoid triggering foods:
   Nuts, chocolate, acidic fruits, or foods patient identifies by experience

Avoid trauma:
   Toothbrush trauma, cheek bite, etc

Avoid stress:
   Now that is useless advice... who has the time to avoid stress?

Avoid sodium lauryl sulfate:
   A soap found in most toothpaste and mouthwashes. Consider Biotene Dry Mouth toothpaste.

Consider an antimicrobial mouthrinse:
   Chlorhexidine Gluconate (Rx on page 72) or **Listerine.** For prevention only. Do not prescribe for treatment – it does not work to treat lesion and the alcohol stings.

APHTHOUS ULCERS (CANKER SORES) MANAGEMENT

PAIN RELIEF

Products which coat the lesion or numb the ulcers or do both:

Coat and numb lesion:
Orabase
Zilactin
Kank-A

Coat lesion only:
Liquid Carafate
Canker Cover

Coat the surface of ulcers: various brands available

PHARMACOLOGICAL TREATMENT

Corticosteroids to reverse the autoimmune process (all are by prescription):

Triamcinolone paste (often not potent enough) (Rx page 58)

Fluocinonide ointment (formerly Lidex) (Rx page 58)

Clobetasol ointment (Temovate) (Rx page 58)

Dexamethasone elixir (Rx page 59)

On rare occasions, use **Prednisone** (oral), 40 mg/day for 7 days (Rx page 59)

Cauterizing (Chemical) Treatment:

Sulfonated Phenolics and Sulfuric Acid (Debacterol) (Rx page 60)

(ACUTE) NECROTIZING ULCERATING GINGIVITIS (ANUG OR NUG)

NUG is a specific bacterial (spirochetal) infection.

TREATMENT STEPS:

1. **Hydrogen peroxide** rinse and/or warm saline rinse

2. **Chlorhexidine Gluconate** (Rx page 72) or **Povidone-Iodine** (Betadine) to aid in treating infection

3. **Clindamycin** or **Metronidazole** to treat infection (Rx pages 38 to 39)

4. Short-term pain medication as needed (pages 21 to 32)

5. Dental cleaning when patient is comfortable

Rx	**Povidone-Iodine** (Betadine) **10% solution**
Disp	8 oz
Sig	Rinse 1 teaspoonful in mouth for 1 minute and expectorate, 2 times per day

> **NOTE:** Not to be used in patients allergic to iodine. Solution should be completely expectorated (*it tastes awful, they will want to spit it all out*). For short-term use only, maximum: 2 days.

MEDICATIONS: ORAL ALLERGY

Rx   **Cetirizine** (ZyrTEC) **10 mg**

Disp   16 tablets

Sig   5 to 10 mg once a day

> **NOTE:** Effective antihistamine, less sedation, safer and more convenient than Benadryl.

MEDICATIONS: ORAL AUTOIMMUNE DISEASE

Rx	**Fluocinonide ointment* 0.05%** (formerly Lidex)
Disp	15 g
Sig	Apply thin layer to oral lesions 2 to 4 times per day

Rx	**Clobetasol** (Temovate) **ointment* 0.05%**
Disp	15 g
Sig	Apply thin layer to oral lesions twice daily for up to 2 weeks (maximum dose: 50 g/week); discontinue application when control is achieved; if no improvement is seen, reassessment of diagnosis may be necessary

Rx	**Triamcinolone paste 0.1%**
Disp	5 g
Sig	Apply thin layer to affected area 3 times per day. Press a small dab (about ¼ inch) to the lesion until a thin film develops; a larger quantity may be required for coverage of some lesions. For optimal results, use only enough to coat the lesion with a thin film; do not rub in.

NOTE: If stronger corticosteroid is needed, use Fluocinonide

*NOTE: Label on the tube of these products will say "for external use only." Use in mouth is considered "off-label." These drugs have been and are used safely, as directed, on oral mucosa for oral inflammatory/autoimmune diseases. Patient should be informed of off-label use.

MEDICATIONS: ORAL AUTOIMMUNE DISEASE

Rx	**Dexamethasone elixir 0.5 mg/5 mL**
Disp	500 mL
Sig	Rinse with 5 mL for 2 minutes 4 times/day and expectorate

Rx	**Prednisone 5 mg**
Disp	40 tablets
Sig	Take 4 tablets in AM and 4 tablets at noon for 5 days

CAUTION:
1. Take medication with food.
2. Use with extreme caution. This is a potent systemic dosage. Consult with patient's physician, an oral medicine dentist (at dental schools), *Lexicomp Online for Dentistry* (https://store.wolterskluwercdi.com/CDI), or *Drug Information Handbook for Dentistry,* if questions on dosage, indications, or contraindications arise.

MEDICATIONS: APHTHOUS (CAUTERIZER)

Rx **Sulfonated Phenolics and Sulfuric Acid** (Debacterol)

Disp   1 tube

Sig   Break internal glass tube, touch saturated cotton tip to thoroughly dried ulcer (warn patient, ***it will hurt!***). Hold in place for 5 to 1 seconds.

> INGREDIENT: Sulfonated phenolics 50% and sulfuric acid 30%
>
> **NOTE:** Not recommended to apply more than 1 treatment each ulcer; if ulcer persists, reconsider diagnosis, may not be a canker sore.

ANGULAR CHEILITIS
(CRACKING IN THE CORNER OF THE MOUTH)

Rx **Nystatin and Triamcinolone cream** (formerly Mycolog-II)

Disp   15 g

Sig   Apply sparingly to corners of mouth 2 to 4 times/day. Therapy should be discontinued when control is achieved; if no improvement is seen, reassessment of diagnosis may be necessary

> INGREDIENT: Nystatin 100,000 units and triamcinolone acetonide 0.1%

MAGIC MOUTHWASH

Clinicians and patients are convinced that *their* Magic Mouthwash is great for use in a specific application. However, an investigation of this "product" (*Pharmacist's Letter*) reveals that there is no specific formulation for Magic Mouthwash. Most formulations contain viscous lidocaine or diphenhydramine for analgesia and Maalox, Milk of Magnesia, sucralfate, or a similar antacid to coat the surface of the mucosa. The other ingredients are an antibiotic (tetracycline) to reduce bacterial flora around the lesion, though other mechanisms of action have been postulated, and/or an antifungal (nystatin) to stop fungal growth, and/or corticosteroid (hydrocortisone, dexamethasone) to reduce inflammation. The usual instructions are to use every 4 to 6 hours, hold in mouth for 1 to 2 minutes, then expectorate. Patients should be instructed to shake bottle well before using and not to eat or drink for 30 minutes after use.

Here is a good example of a magic mouthwash*:

Viscous lidocaine 2%	150 mL
Diphenhydramine 12.5 mg/5 mL	20 mL
Hydrocortisone (Solu-Cortef)	100 mg
Tetracycline or Doxycycline	2 g
Nystatin suspension	20 mL

Swish and expectorate 15 to 30 mL every 4 to 6 hours

Alternatively, here is a good example of a magic mouthwash without steroids*:

Viscous lidocaine 2%	1 part
Diphenhydramine 12.5 mg/5 mL	1 part
Maalox	1 part

Swish 5 mL, hold and expectorate; repeat no more than every 4 hours

The pharmacist needs detailed instructions to formulate the correct rinse; just writing for "Magic Mouthwash" is not specific enough.

7) MISCELLANEOUS

Dentin Hypersensitivity*

Anticaries Agents*

Antiplaque / Antigingivitis Agents*

Halitosis / Oral Malodor

Probiotics, Prebiotics, and Oral Health

Necrotizing Ulcerating Periodontitis
  (HIV-associated Periodontal Disease)

Muscle Relaxants

Periodontal Disease

Salivary Problems

Sinus Infection Treatment

Dry Socket

Pediatric Oral Dosages

---

*NOTE: Check https://www.ada.org/en/science-research/ada-seal-of-acceptance/ada-seal-shopping-list for most current list of over-the-counter consumer products that have the ADA Seal of Acceptance.

DENTIN HYPERSENSITIVITY

SUGGESTED STEPS IN RESOLVING DENTIN HYPERSENSITIVITY:

A thorough exam to rule out any other source for the problem such as tooth fracture, occlusal trauma, or irreversible pulpitis, must be done first. The most common reason for persistent hypersensitivity is bruxing.

TREATMENT STEPS: Start with Step 1. Progress through steps as needed, until hypersensitivity is controlled.

Step 1. **Home treatment** with a desensitizing toothpaste containing potassium nitrate (or stannous fluoride) (used to brush teeth at least 2 times per day, as well as a thin layer applied to affected teeth and left overnight, each night for 3 to 4 weeks). Tell patient not to use tartar control toothpaste. It may slow natural occlusion of dentinal tubules by preventing calcium precipitation.

Step 2. **In office**, apply glutaraldehyde/HEMA preparation to exposed root surface (eg, Glu/Sense, GLUMA Comfort Bond & Desensitizer).

Step 3. Apply potassium nitrate-based toothpaste in a bleaching tray for 10 to 30 minutes a day as needed.

NOTE: This is the best way to prevent bleaching sensitivity.

Step 4. Coat exposed root surface with light cured self-etching resin (eg, Clearfil SE Bond 2, Clearfil SE Protect Bond).

Potassium nitrate is the active ingredient in all FDA-approved desensitizing toothpastes (**Crest Sensitivity Protection**, **Sensodyne**, **Colgate Sensitive**, **Oragel Sensitive**, etc), except **Crest ProHealth** which contains stannous fluoride.

NOTE: Check the ADA website https://www.ada.org/en/science-research/ada-seal-of-acceptance/ada-seal-shopping-list for current listing of ADA-accepted consumer products.

ANTICARIES AGENTS

MANAGING DENTAL CARIES AS A DISEASE

The cause and mechanism of dental caries is well understood, yet there is not yet consensus on caries management as new treatments continue to evolve. In September 2011, an ADA expert panel evaluated the existing evidence for caries prevention. Dietary improvement (decreased exposure to fermentable carbohydrates/sugar), topical fluorides, and sealants have the highest levels of evidence for caries prevention and should be used first.

If these are not enough, only 2 adjunctive modalities, Xylitol and Chlorhexidine-Thymol varnish, had adequate science and expert opinion support to recommend them (Nonfluoride Caries – Preventive Agents: Executive Summary of Evidence-Based Clinical Recommendations, ADA Expert Panel. *JADA.* 2011;142(9):1065-1071).

A more recent randomized clinical trial demonstrated beneficial effects using topical fluoride and 0.12% chlorhexidine gluconate rinse based upon bacterial challenge (A Randomized Clinical Trial of Anticaries Therapies Targeted according to Risk Assessment [Caries Management by Risk Assessment]. *Caries Res.* 2012;46(2):118-129).

Recent literature supports the value of Caries Risk Assessment tools (How useful are current caries risk assessment tools in informing the oral health care decision making process, *JADA.* 2019;150(2):91-102). Recent literature also confirms limiting the intake of fermentable carbohydrate, the aggressive use of fluoride in all forms, plus, in extreme risk categories, chlorhexidine mouthrinse to kill bacteria and baking soda mouthrinse to neutralize acid are the best current caries management modalities (Caries Management by Risk Assessment (CAMBRA): An update for use in clinical practice for patients aged 6 through adult. *CDAJ.* 2019;47(1):25-34.) In extreme risk categories, minimally invasive restorative procedures and silver diamide fluoride is also recommended.

A key part of any caries management strategy is patient education. A caries risk assessment form filled out with the patient, so they understand the causes and prevention of decay, is crucial to motivating compliance and getting a long-term positive result.

ANTICARIES AGENTS

XYLITOL: Xylitol is a natural sugar that cariogenic bacteria cannot metabolize into tooth-dissolving acidic by-products. Its presence alters the oral bacterial environment and decreases the risk of decay (https://www.aapd.org/research/oral-health-policies--recommendations/use-of-xylitol/).

> DOSAGE: Chew 2 sticks of gum for 5 to 10 minutes, 3 to 4 times day (discontinue use if TMJ symptoms occur) or suck on xylitol candy (6 to 10 g/day, spread throughout the day).
>
> **NOTE:** Not for children 5 years or younger, due to risk of choking.
>
> SOURCES: www.xlear.com, www.epicdental.com, and other brands.

CHLORHEXIDINE-THYMOL VARNISH: 1:1 mixture is useful for root caries, presumably by killing the cariogenic bacteria responsible for decay. (See also chlorhexidine gluconate oral rinse on page 72).

> DOSAGE: Apply layer of varnish to roots every 3 months (in-office procedure).
>
> **NOTE:** There is not good evidence to support the use of this combination or any concentration of chlorhexidine alone for the control of coronal caries.
>
> SOURCES: Cervitec Plus, www.ivoclarvivadent.com

– also –

Consider the CariFree System® – information at www.carifree.com
They focus on caries and have designed a scientific anticaries system for clinical practice, including caries risk assessment, bacterial load measurement, and a complete product line focused on pH, biofilm modification, and remineralization

ANTICARIES AGENTS

SILVER DIAMINE FLUORIDE 38%: Silver diamine Fluoride is the newest old thing we have in dentistry. We still have it, because it works. It stops dental decay in its tracks. The reason we stopped using it and some people will never start, is because it turns decay black. Very few people want black teeth. But children with extensive decay in baby teeth* and seniors with decay in posterior cervical areas or at the margins of posterior crowns, don't care about black, they just want decay stopped, so Silver diamine fluoride definitely has an important place in the management of dental decay. Once the decay is stopped and the teeth harden, the black can be masked with composite, or more compatible glass ionomer, if desired.

The brand, Advantage Arrest, is the only FDA approved source for silver diamine fluoride in the US, at this point. 877-684-4858 or https://www.elevateoralcare.com/products/AdvantageArrest.

As a note, FDA has approved silver diamine fluoride for the management of hypersensitivity. Its use as an anticaries treatment is, "off label", but is a well established and easily documented, off label use.

Crystal YO, Marghalani AA, Ureles SD, et al. Use of silver diamine fluoride for dental caries management in children and adolescents, including those with special health care needs. *Pediatr Dent.* 2017;39(5):E135-E145.

http://www.aapd.org/media/policies_guidelines/p_silverdiamine.pdf

Clayton RL, Urquhart O, Araujo MWB, et al. Evidence-based clinical practice guideline on nonrestorative treatments for carious lesions: A report from the American Dental Association. *J Am Dent Assoc.* 2018;149(10):837-849.e19. doi:10.1016/j.adaj.2018.07.002

ANTICARIES AGENTS

Fluorides to "harden" tooth structure*:

Of course, OTC toothpaste (1,000 to 1,500 ppm) and consider OTC fluoride rinses (230 ppm)

High Caries Rate:

Rx: Sodium fluoride (5,000 ppm) gel or toothpaste
and
Fluoride varnish (22,600 ppm) applied every 6 months

*See ADA topical fluoride guidelines – http://ebd.ada.org/~/media/EBD/Files/JADA_updated_executive_summary_Nov_2013.ashx

http://www.aapd.org/media/Policies_Guidelines/P_FluorideUse.pdf

FLUORIDE: PRESCRIPTION SYSTEMIC

Rx	**Sodium Fluoride tablets** (tablet size based on table below*)
Disp	120 tablets
Sig	Chew and dissolve 1 tablet in mouth, swish, then swallow, once per day, preferably before bedtime after brushing

> **NOTE:** Chewing and swishing the fluoride in mouth is very important. Much of the protective effects are topical
> *1 mg of fluoride equals 2.2 mg of sodium fluoride

ADA Recommended Supplemental Fluoride Dosage Schedule

Age (years)	Concentration of fluoride ion in drinking water (ppm)		
	<0.3	0.3 to 0.6	>0.6
6 mo to 3 y	0.25 mg	0	0
3 to 6 y	0.5 mg	0.25 mg	0
6 to 16 y	1 mg	0.5 mg	0

ANTICARIES AGENTS

FLUORIDE: PRESCRIPTION TOPICAL

Rx **Neutral Sodium Fluoride gel / toothpaste 1.1** (5,000 ppm)

Disp 2 oz

Sig Brush on teeth or place 1 teaspoonful of gel in fluoride tray and apply to teeth for 3 to 5 minutes, or while you are in the shower, once per day

COMMERCIAL PRODUCTS:
- Clinpro 5000
- FluoriMax 5000 (Elevate Care)
- Neutracare Home Topical (Oral-B)
- PreviDent Gel or Toothpaste (Colgate)
- Many other brands, all are effective

Rx **Fluoride varnish** (22,600 ppm F)

COMMERCIAL PRODUCTS FOR DENTAL OFFICE:
- Vanish (3M)
- Duraphat (Colgate)
- FluoriMax 2.5% NaF Varnish (Elevate Care)
- PreviDent Varnish
- Many other brands, all are effective

ANTICARIES AGENTS

FLUORIDE: NONPRESCRIPTION TOPICAL

Rx   Any **ADA-Approved toothpaste** (1,000 to 1,500 ppm)

Rx   **OTC Fluoride rinses** (230 ppm F)

    COMMERCIAL PRODUCTS:
        ACT Fluoride Rinse (Johnson & Johnson)
        Fluorigard (Colgate)
        Some of the Listerine rinses

Rx   **Stannous Fluoride 0.4%** (brush on gel) (1,500 ppm)

Disp 4 oz

Sig   Brush on teeth once per day

    COMMERCIAL PRODUCTS:
        Gel-Kam Gel (Colgate)
        PerioMed (3M)
        Omni Gel

ADA ACCEPTED ANTIPLAQUE AND ANTIGINGIVITIS AGENTS

Plaque seems to be the root of all dental/oral health evil, and eliminating it is a constant and elusive destination for hygienists, dentists and patients. The plaque elimination journey gets more challenging for everyone when the plaque starts to calcify.

Most plaque is simply a collection of normal and healthy oral organisms in the wrong place. Their presence, for example, along the marginal gingiva, leads to irritation and then inflammation (gingivitis). At other times, and in some people's mouths and in some oral environments, the organisms populating the plaque can transform and become populated with disease-associated organisms (dysbiosis) leading to periodontitis and/or dental decay.

Plaque removal/plaque control has traditionally been done only two ways. Commonly it is physical removal using brushes and abrasives. Soap and water also fit into this physical approach. Another approach, often used in combination with brushing, is the use of disinfectants such as the Over-the-Counter (OTC) stannous fluoride and/or essential oils or prescription (Rx) chlorhexidine.

A new, effective, and evolving technology for plaque and gingivitis control is the use of modified, food grade safe chelators, most specifically EDTA, similar to, but not the same as what is now used in tartar control toothpastes, to change the local environment at the tooth surface, so plaque is naturally repelled. There is no abrasive and it is not toxic to the healthy oral flora.

Physical removal:
   All toothbrushes, proxy brushes, and floss
   All orally used abrasives in toothpastes, baking soda, charcoal
   Soaps (most commonly, sodium lauryl sulfate) that make toothpaste foam
   Water

Chemical Disinfectants:
   Rx: Chlorhexidine
   OTC: Stannous Fluoride (Crest, Colgate, Parodontax, others)
   Listerine (and generic formulations of the same essential oils)

Chelation:
   OTC: LivFresh Dental Gel (getlivfresh.com)

ADA ACCEPTED ANTIPLAQUE AND ANTIGINGIVITIS AGENTS

Rx	**Chlorhexidine Gluconate oral rinse 0.12%**
Disp	3 x 16 oz (473 mL)
Sig	Floss and brush teeth 2 times per day, completely rinse toothpaste from mouth and swish 15 mL (one capful) undiluted oral rinse around in mouth for 30 seconds, then expectorate. Caution patient not to swallow the medicine and instruct not to eat for 2 to 3 hours after treatment (cap on bottle measures 15 mL).

CAUTION: Chlorhexidine may:
- stain teeth yellow to brown
- alter taste (temporary)
- increase the deposition of calculus
- and requires a prescription

NOTE: Peridex, PerioGard, and other brands
Also, consider for patients with high decay rate (see page 66).

Rx	**Listerine (OTC)**
Disp	To be determined by practitioner
Sig	Rinse 1 tablespoonful in mouth for 30 seconds, 2 times per day

Rx	**Crest ProHealth toothpaste or Colgate Total toothpaste (OTC)**
Disp	To be determined by practitioner
Sig	Brush teeth with toothpaste 2 times per day for 2 minutes

Rx	**LivFresh Dental Gel**
Disp	To be determined by practitioner
Sig	Brush teeth with tooth gel 2 times per day for 2 minutes

HALITOSIS/ORAL MALODOR

Halitosis is a common complaint and is most often associated with bacteria in the oral cavity. There can be other extraoral sources/reasons for the complaint, including medical/systemic problems and even a neurosis or psychosis, halitophobia. As with all successful treatments, halitosis management begins with a correct diagnosis.

Bacteria in the oral cavity is the most common cause (75%) of halitosis, presenting as a coated tongue, periodontal disease, or infection. There are also a variety of systemic causes including diabetes; kidney failure; tonsil abnormalities (eg, tonsilloliths); sinus, upper respiratory, or lung infection; gastric reflux; and cancer, that should be ruled out, especially in persistent and challenging cases. If no obvious odor is detected, but the patient remains very concerned, then halitophobia should be considered and a referral to a clinical psychologist would be appropriate.

Management/Treatment is focused on eliminating the cause, which in most cases is oral bacteria.

1. Decrease oral bacteria

   Brushing of teeth and tongue (back of the tongue, at least to the circumvalate papilla and beyond). If still a problem, a professional cleaning, including scale and root planing, if needed.

   The use of antimicrobial mouthwash and/or toothpaste (suggested active ingredients: chlorhexidine, triclosan, zinc chloride, cetylpyridinium chloride). Mouth rinses without an active antimicrobial ingredient only transiently mask the smell, which can provide some emotional reassurance.

   Interproximal cleaning, like flossing and using toothpicks, can help remove plaque, which can harbor oral bacteria.

HALITOSIS/ORAL MALODOR

2. Eliminate oral odor sources

    Minimize odiferous foods (mostly sulfur-containing foods such as garlic and onions).

    Some people have a unique odor-causing response to milk products or diet sodas.

3. Stay hydrated; dry mouth, for any reason, is conducive to the growth of odor-causing bacteria.

REFERENCES

Avincsal MO, Altundag A, Ulusoy S, Dinc ME, Dalgic A, Topak M. Halitosis associated volatile sulphur compound levels in patients with laryngopharyngeal reflux. *Eur Arch Otohinolaryngol.* 2016;273(6):1515-1520.

Madhushankari GS, Yamunadevi A, Selvamani M, Mohan Kumar KP, Basandi PS Halitosis - an overview: part I - classification, etiology, and pathophysiology of halitosis. *Pharm Bioallied Sci.* 2015;7(Suppl 2):S339-343.

Marsicano JA, de Moura-Grec PG, Bonato RC, Sales-Peres Mde C, Sales-Peres A, Sales-Peres SH. Gastroesophageal reflux, dental erosion, and halitosis in epidemiological surveys a systematic review. *Eur J Gastroenterol Hepatol.* 2013;25(2):135-141.

Porter SR, Scully C. Oral malodor (halitosis). *BMJ.* 2006;333(7569):632-635. Available a https://www.ncbi.nlm.nih.gov/pmc/articles/

PROBIOTICS, PREBIOTICS, AND ORAL HEALTH

One of the newest areas of "Dental Pharmacology" is managing/altering the oral flora to improve/maintain oral health. Probiotics are the "good" organisms that are known to live in a healthy mouth. Prebiotics are the food/special compounds/saccharides (sugars)/polysaccharides that good organisms need to survive and grow.

How the good organisms work to establish and maintain oral health is an active area of research with many hypotheses. Theories include that the good organisms either out-compete or actively destroy the bad organisms.

Lactobacillus and bifidobacteria (found in most yogurt) are the most well known probiotics. There is limited evidence that these organisms may have a positive impact on caries control, by competing against cariogenic streptococci. There are no specifically formulated dental products with these organisms.

At this point, there is much research to be done. Science has not yet identified all the bad and good organisms in the oral cavity and how each organism impacts oral health.

Based on that, the use of probiotics and prebiotics should be considered as adjuncts to proven therapies and their use should be considered only after, or in conjunction with, established treatments for oral problems like caries and periodontal disease.

PROBIOTICS, PREBIOTICS, AND ORAL HEALTH

Probiotics

Probiotics are defined by the Food and Agriculture Organization of the World Health Organization as live microorganisms that, when administered in adequate amounts, confer a health benefit on the host by improving its intestinal microbial balance.

ProBiora 3 (ProBiora Health): contains *S. oralis*, *S. uberis*, *S. rattus*; https://probiorahealth.com

PRO-Dental by Hyperbiotics: contains *S. salivaris* M18 and K12; https://www.hyperbiotics.com

TheraBreath Oral Care Probiotics by TheraBreath: contains *S. salivaris* M18 and K12; https://www.therabreath.com

Prebiotics

Prebiotics have been defined as nondigestible food ingredients that beneficially affect the host by selectively stimulating the growth and/or activity of one or a limited number of bacteria in the colon.

Isothrive

Prebiotin

REFERENCES

Allaker RP, Ian Douglas CW. Non-conventional therapies for oral infections. *Virulence* 2015;6(3):196-207. Available at http://www.tandfonline.com/doi/full/10.4161/21505594.2014.983783?src=recsys

MANAGEMENT OF NECROTIZING ULCERATING PERIODONTITIS
(HIV-Associated Periodontal Disease)

INITIAL TREATMENT (IN-OFFICE)

- Povidone-Iodine (Betadine) rinse (page 56)

  NOTE: Ensure patient has no iodine allergies

- Gentle debridement / dental cleaning

AT-HOME

- Chlorhexidine rinse (page 72)
- Metronidazole (Flagyl) 7 to 10 days (page 39)

FOLLOW-UP THERAPY

- Proper dental cleaning including scaling and root planing (repeat as needed)
- Continue Chlorhexidine rinse as needed

NOTE: Most patients respond well to therapy and only normal oral hygiene and cleaning are needed.

MUSCLE RELAXANTS

Muscle relaxants can be of some small value, sometimes for "TMJ" problem (myofascial pain dysfunction problems). Muscle relaxants are of no value pain is exclusively localized in the joint. Besides the fact that muscle relaxant seldom help, they have one major drawback, they relax ALL the muscles, no just the jaw muscles. Patients often feel unusually weak and tired, adding t their general level of distress – warn the patient about such concerns. Th drugs suggested below are only for short-term use (maximum: 3 weeks). N response in that time means they are not effective and should be discontinued If the patient responds, a refill can be considered, but both drugs below hav more side effects, dependence, and drug interactions the longer they are use

Rx	**Clonazepam 0.5 mg**
Disp	40 tablets
Sig	Take 1 tablet before sleep (if response is minimal and there hav been no unwanted side effects after 3 days, then an addition: 1 tablet can be added in the morning)

    NOTE: Not to be used in elderly; severe risk of falling.

Rx	**Cyclobenzaprine 5 mg** (formerly Flexeril)
Disp	40 tablets
Sig	Initial: 5 mg 3 times/day; may increase to 7.5 to 10 mg 3 time day if needed

    NOTE: Not to be used in elderly; severe risk of falling.

                It is important to review the package insert especia for information about contraindications, side effect and precautions.

PERIODONTAL DISEASE

The mechanism of bone loss in periodontal disease is not fully understood, but if the patient has good to reasonable professional and home care, and is still losing bone, doxycycline may be of value. The low dose used is not considered antimicrobial, but inhibits collagenase/metalloproteinases, enzymes associated with inflammation, that contribute to bone loss.

It is appropriate to discuss this medical approach to managing periodontal disease with your periodontist, to get their perspective on patient selection and efficacy.*

Rx	**Doxycycline 20 mg**
Disp	180 tablets
Sig	Take 1 tablet 2 times per day

NOTE: Do not use during pregnancy.

Some patients will cut a 100 mg tablet of doxycycline in quarters (but you need a dexterous patient).

Periostat is a branded formulation of doxycycline, 20 mg, available in Canada.

*The duration of treatment is 1 to 3 years.

SALIVARY HYPOSECRETION / XEROSTOMIA

Dry mouth is most commonly a side effect of medications, but can be caused by radiation (cancer treatment) or immunologic (Sjögren's Syndrome) destruction of the salivary glands. Advanced age can also lead to decreased resting levels of saliva production, though stimulated flows are usually normal.

TREATMENT: If salivary glands are still functional, they can be stimulated with pilocarpine or cevimeline.

Rx	**Pilocarpine hydrochloride** (Salagen) **5 mg**
Disp	90 tablets
Sig	Take 1 to 2 tablets 3 to 4 times per day (maximum dose: 10 mg 3 times per day)

 CAUTION: Read prescribing information. Many contraindications (ie, asthma, glaucoma, severe hepatic impairment) and precautions (eye, heart, lung, and other diseases)

 NOTE: Pilocarpine is available as a generic; minimum 90-day therapy required for optimum effects, so adjust amount dispensed accordingly.

Rx	**Cevimeline** (Evoxac) **30 mg**
Disp	90 capsules
Sig	Take 1 capsule 3 times per day

 CAUTION: Read prescribing information. Many contraindications (ie, glaucoma, asthma) and precautions (eye, heart, lung, and other diseases).

SALIVARY HYPOSECRETION / XEROSTOMIA

PALLIATIVE TREATMENT OF DRY MOUTH:

Artificial Lubricant:

    Biotene Dry Mouth Oral Balance Gel (GSK)

    Biotene Dry Mouth Oral Rinse or Moisturizing Spray (GSK)
    (https://dental-professional.com/Products/Biotene.html)

Artificial Salivas:

    Saliva substitute (3M)

    Mouth Kote (Pasnell)

    Moi-Stir (Pendopharm)

    Most people just use plain water in a small squirt bottle

Nonirritating Toothpaste:

    Biotene Dry Mouth Toothpaste (GSK)

Mouth Lozenges:

    Salese with Xylitol (http://nuvorainc.com)

NOTE: The Sjögren's foundation (www.sjogrens.org) is the best source for you and your patient on dry mouth management – no matter why they have dry mouth. They publish the *Moisture Seekers Newsletter*.

See "Managing Dental Caries as a Disease" for those patients with severe xerostomia (page 65).

Water:

    Some people just keep a spray bottle of water with them. It is inexpensive and provides about the same amount of benefit and relief.

SALIVARY HYPERSECRETION (SIALORRHEA)

The drug below can be used to block excessive salivary flow during restorative procedures. Propantheline can have a variety of unpleasant side effects like blurred vision, stomach upset, decreased sweating, and others. Patients should be warned so they are aware and are not surprised or distressed.

Rx	**Propantheline 15 mg**
Disp	# (Tablet quantity determined by number of appointments needed)
Sig	Take 1 tablet 30 minutes before dental appointment

CAUTION: Read prescribing information. Many contraindications such as glaucoma, ulcerative colitis, and myasthenia gravis. Can cause dry eyes, so remove contact lenses.

NOTE: In some patients, 2 tablets may be needed.

SINUS INFECTION TREATMENT

Dentist may elect to treat sinuses, but only to rule out dental problems. If the patient has no dental complaints, refer to physician.

Rx	**Amoxicillin 500 mg**
Disp	21 tablets
Sig	Take 1 tablet 3 times per day

– OR –

Rx	**Amoxicillin and Clavulanate** (Augmentin) **500/125 mg**
Disp	30 tablets
Sig	Take 1 tablet 3 times per day
	INGREDIENTS: Amoxicillin 500 mg and Clavulanate Potassium 125 mg

TREATMENT: The selected antibiotic (above) should be used with the compounds below, which block the swelling effect of histamine (Claritin) and shrink the sinuses.

Rx	**Loratadine** (Claritin) **10 mg (OTC)**
Disp	14 tablets
Sig	Take 1 tablet per day

Rx	**Oxymetazoline (Nasal)**
Disp	15 mL
Sig	2 to 3 sprays in each nostril twice daily for up to 3 days
	BRANDS: Afrin Nasal Spray, Mucinex Nasal Spray Moisture, Vicks Sinex Moisturizing, various other brands

DRY SOCKET (ACUTE / ALVEOLAR OSTEITIS)

This is a necrosis of bone following a dental extraction. It is usually caused by the loss of the blood clot within the extraction site, so the area has to heal by secondary intention. It is not an infection and usually not associated with an infection. Treatment is designed to soothe the pain while the area heals.

TREATMENT:

1. Gently irrigate socket with saline.

2. Gently fill socket site with iodoform gauze coated with a gel of local anesthetic and eugenol (Sultan and other brands; Alvogyl by Septodont is available in Canada, but does not have FDA approval).

3. Remove gauze after 2 days (Alvogyl dissolves on its own, and does not need to be removed).

4. Repeat application if pain persists.

NOTE: Prescribe pain medication as needed (pages 21 to 32).

If obvious pus/infection, then it is not a dry socket, it is an infection and you must manage as an infection and prescribe antibiotics (pages 33 to 39).

If problem persists, especially if pain is not severe, and patient takes bone-antiresorptive drugs, such as bisphosphonates, consider possibility of antiresorptive agent-induced osteonecrosis (pages 101 to 102).

PEDIATRIC ORAL DOSAGES

Pediatric dosages are given as mg of drug per kg (1 kg = 2.2 lbs) of child per 24 hours. **The child dose should never exceed the adult dose**, even if the calculation suggests it does.

The table on the following pages lists the <u>maximum oral dose in mg/kg (1 kg = 2.2 lbs) for a child in a 24-hour period</u>. It also indicates the frequency of dosing. Please note the maximum 24-hour dose must be divided by the suggested number of doses per 24 hours, to get the amount for each dose.

If there are any concerns or questions as to appropriateness of dosage, drug interactions, or indications for the drug, consult the child's physician, pharmacist, or the drug's package insert information.

NOTE: **In California, and possibly other states (check your state law)**, Oral sedation means anything given by mouth that will sedate or relax the child. This would include sedative/hypnotics (benzodiazepines, barbiturates), antihistamines, opioids, and chloral hydrate.

PEDIATRIC ORAL DOSAGES

DRUG	INDICATION	DOSAGE
Acetaminophen	Analgesia	10 to 15 mg/kg/dose every 4 to 6 hours as needed; do not exceed 5 doses in 24 hours; maximum daily dose: 75 mg/kg/day not to exceed 4 g/24 hours
Acetaminophen 120 mg + Codeine 12 mg/5 mL or Acetaminophen 300 mg + Codeine 15 mg	Analgesia	>12 years: Codeine component: 0.5 to 1 mg/kg/dose every 4 to 6 hours (maximum: codeine 60 mg/dose and acetaminophen 4 g/24 hours)
Acyclovir	Treatment of initial episodes of herpes simplex infection	20 mg/kg/dose 4 times daily for 5 to 7 days (maximum: 800 mg/dose)
Amoxicillin	Bacterial infection	20 to 100 mg/kg/day in divided doses every 8 hours (maximum dose: 875 mg/dose)
Azithromycin	Bacterial infection, penicillin allergy	10 to 12 mg/kg/dose on day 1 (usual maximum dose: 500 mg/dose) followed by 5 to 6 mg/kg once daily (usual maximum dose: 250 mg/dose)
Cephalexin	Bacterial infection	25 to 100 mg/kg/day divided every 6 to 12 hours (maximum: 4 g/24 hours)
Clindamycin	Bacterial infection, penicillin allergy	8 to 40 mg/kg/day divided in 3 to 4 equally divided doses (maximum daily dose: 1,800 mg/24 hours)
Clotrimazole	Oropharyngeal candidiasis	≥3 years: 10 mg troche dissolved slowly 5 times/day

(continue

PEDIATRIC ORAL DOSAGES

(continued)

DRUG	INDICATION	DOSAGE
Diazepam*	Anxiolysis	Infants ≥6 months and Adolescents: 0.2 to 0.3 mg/kg (maximum dose: 10 mg) 45 to 60 minutes prior to procedure; Children: 0.2 to 0.5 mg/kg (maximum dose: 10 mg) 45 to 60 minutes prior to procedure
Fluconazole	Oropharyngeal candidiasis	Initial: 6 mg/kg/dose on day 1, followed by 3 to 6 mg/kg/dose once daily (usual adult dose: 100 to 200 mg/24 hours) (non-HIV patients)
Hydroxyzine*	Anxiolysis	<6 years: 50 mg/day in 4 divided doses; ≥6 years; 50 to 100 mg/day in 4 divided doses
Ibuprofen	Analgesia	<50 kg: 4 to 10 mg/kg/dose every 6 to 8 hours (maximum single dose: 400 mg; maximum daily dose: 40 mg/kg/24 hours); ≥50 kg: Refer to adult dosing
Metronidazole	Bacterial infection	15 to 50 mg/kg/day in divided doses every 8 hours (maximum dose: 2,250 mg/24 hours)
Naproxen	Analgesia	Children and Adolescents <60 kg: Limited data available: Oral: 5 to 6 mg/kg/dose every 12 hours (maximum daily dose: 1 g/day (Berde 2002); doses as high as 10 mg/kg/dose have also been recommended (APS 2008)) Children and Adolescents ≥60 kg: Limited data available: Oral: 250 to 375 mg twice daily; maximum daily dose: 1,000 mg/day (Berde 2002)

See **Note** on page 85.

NOTE: For pediatric doses for the prophylaxis of infectious (bacterial) endocarditis, see pages 90 to 95.

8) MANAGING MEDICALLY COMPLEX PATIENTS

Prophylactic Antibiotic Coverage

Prevention of Orthopaedic Implant Infection

Antiresorptive Agent-Induced Osteonecrosis of the Jaw

Pregnant and Breastfeeding Patients

PROPHYLACTIC ANTIBIOTIC COVERAGE

A. Prevention of Bacterial Endocarditis

B. Prevention of Prosthetic Joint Infections

C. Other Medical Conditions

The following cardiac and artificial joint guidelines are the only official ADA sanctioned guidelines for prophylactic antibiotic use in dentistry. No others exist as of the printing of this booklet.

A literature review (Little JW, Falace DA, Miller CS, and Rhodus NL. "Antibiotic Prophylaxis in Dentistry: An Update," *Gen Dent*, 2008 56(1):20-28) suggests that the below listed medical situations may warrant prophylactic antibiotic coverage for dental procedures, but there are no official guidelines to do so.

1. Dental treatment of:

    Immunosuppressed patients (neutropenia <1,000 and/or CD4 <200 cells/microL)

    Poorly controlled type 1 diabetic patients

    Poorly controlled organ transplant patients

    Patients post splenectomy within last 6 months

2. Incisions/manipulation of a dental abscess in patients with a nonvalvular cardiac device.

If you do elect to prophylax in the above situations, the drugs of choice are those suggested for heart and joint prophylaxis. If infection persists/ensues consultation with, or referral to, an oral-maxillofacial surgeon, endodontist, periodontist, or physician, relative to management, is appropriate.

PROPHYLACTIC ANTIBIOTIC COVERAGE FOR THE PREVENTION OF BACTERIAL ENDOCARDITIS

Current American Heart Association Guidelines
Published May 18, 2021, *Circulation,* 143(20):e963-e978.
(https://www.ahajournals.org/doi/10.1161/CIR.0000000000000969)

Cardiac Conditions for Which Prophylaxis for Dental Procedures is Recommended[1,2]

1. Prosthetic cardiac valves, including transcatheter-implanted prostheses and homografts.

2. Prosthetic material used for heart valve repair, such as annuloplasty rings, chords, or clips.

3. Previous Infective Endocarditis

4. Unrepaired cyanotic congenital heart defect (birth defects with oxygen levels lower than normal) or repaired congenital heart defect, with residual shunts or valvular regurgitation at the site adjacent to the site of a prosthetic patch or prosthetic device.

5. Cardiac transplant with valve regurgitation due to a structurally abnormal valve.

If patient's physician requests prophylaxis for dental procedure, but patient does not meet ADA/AHA criteria for needing it, then physician should prescribe prophylaxis, patient takes it under their direction, and they come to you safe for dental procedures.

Except for the cardiac conditions listed above, antibiotic prophylaxis is no longer recommended for any other cardiac condition or problem.

If patient has one of the above cardiac conditions, they need prophylaxis for all dental procedures that bleed or could bleed.

PROPHYLACTIC ANTIBIOTIC COVERAGE FOR THE PREVENTION OF BACTERIAL ENDOCARDITIS

STANDARD REGIMEN

Rx	**Amoxicillin 500 mg**
Disp	4 tablets
Sig	Take 4 tablets (2 g) 30 to 60 minutes before procedure

NOTE: 1) Children 50 mg/kg 30 to 60 minutes before procedure (do not exceed adult dose)

2) No second dose is required for adults or children

STANDARD REGIMEN FOR PATIENTS ALLERGIC TO AMOXICILLIN OR PENICILLIN

Rx	**Cephalexin* 500 mg**
Disp	4 tablets
Sig	Take 4 tablets (2 g) 30 to 60 minutes before procedure

Children >1 year: 50 mg/kg 30 to 60 minutes before procedure (do not exceed adult dose)

– OR –

*Cephalosporins should not be used in individuals with immediate-type hypersensitivity reaction (urticaria, angioedema, or anaphylaxis) to penicill

PROPHYLACTIC ANTIBIOTIC COVERAGE FOR THE PREVENTION OF BACTERIAL ENDOCARDITIS

STANDARD REGIMEN FOR PATIENTS ALLERGIC TO AMOXICILLIN OR PENICILLIN *(continued)*

Rx	**Azithromycin 500 mg**
Disp	1 tablet
Sig	Take 1 tablet (500 mg) 30 to 60 minutes before procedure
	Children: 15 mg/kg 30 to 60 minutes before procedure (do not exceed adult dose)
	Adolescents ≥16 years: 500 mg 30 to 60 minutes before procedure

– OR –

Rx	**Clarithromycin 250 mg**
Disp	2 tablets
Sig	Take 2 tablets (500 mg) 30 to 60 minutes before procedure
	Children: 15 mg/kg 30 to 60 minutes before procedure (do not exceed adult dose)

NOTE: Clindamycin is no longer recommended for antibiotic prophylaxis for a dental procedure.

PROPHYLACTIC ANTIBIOTIC COVERAGE FOR THE PREVENTION OF BACTERIAL ENDOCARDITIS

FOR PATIENTS UNABLE TO TAKE ORAL MEDICATION

Rx **Ampicillin**

2 g IV or IM within 30 to 60 minutes before procedure

Children: 50 mg/kg IV or IM within 30 to 60 minutes before procedure (do not exceed adult dose)

– OR –

Rx **Cefazolin* – *OR* – Ceftriaxone***

1 g IV or IM within 30 to 60 minutes before procedure

Children: 50 mg/kg IV or IM within 30 to 60 minutes before procedure (do not exceed adult dose)

*Cephalosporins should not be used in individuals with immediate-type hypersensitivity reaction (urticaria, angioedema, or anaphylaxis) to penicillin

PROPHYLACTIC ANTIBIOTIC COVERAGE FOR THE PREVENTION OF BACTERIAL ENDOCARDITIS

FOR PATIENTS UNABLE TO TAKE ORAL MEDICATION AND ALLERGIC TO AMPICILLIN, AMOXICILLIN, AND/OR PENICILLIN

Rx   **Cefazolin* – *OR* – Ceftriaxone***

1 g IV or IM within 30 to 60 minutes before procedure

Children: 50 mg/kg IV or IM within 30 to 60 minutes before procedure (do not exceed adult dose)

*Cephalosporins should not be used in individuals with immediate-type hypersensitivity reaction (urticaria, angioedema, or anaphylaxis) to penicillin.

Patients should receive prophylactic antibiotic therapy if they meet the criteria for a specified procedure/condition listed below **and** they have a high-risk cardiovascular condition (listed on page 91).[1]

PROPHYLAXIS RECOMMENDED

All invasive manipulations of the gingival or periapical region or perforation of oral mucosa (includes biopsies, suture removal, placement of orthodontic bands)

PROPHYLAXIS NOT RECOMMENDED

Anesthetic injections through noninfected tissue, radiographs, placement/adjustment/removal of prosthodontics/orthodontic appliances or brackets, shedding of deciduous teeth, trauma-induced bleeding from lips, gums, or oral mucosa

Source: AHA Guidelines

PREVENTION OF ORTHOPAEDIC IMPLANT INFECTION IN PATIENTS UNDERGOING DENTAL PROCEDURE

The American Dental Association and the Council on Scientific Affairs, in January of 2015, provided Clinical Recommendations relative to the Management of Patients with Prosthetic Joints Undergoing Dental Procedures (Sollecito 2015).

The primary recommendation:

In general, for patients with prosthetic joint implants, prophylactic antibiotics are **not recommended** prior to dental procedures to prevent prosthetic joint infections.

The 2015 ADA clinical practice guideline is valid and should continue to inform clinical decisions for dental patients in ambulatory settings. The guideline states clearly that the "evidence fails to demonstrate an association between dental procedures and Prosthetic Joint Infections (PJI) or any effectiveness for any antibiotic prophylaxis." Given this information in conjunction with the potential harm from antibiotic use, using antibiotics before dental procedures is not recommended to prevent PJI.

In February 2017, a joint committee of ADA members and American Association of Orthopedic Surgeons (AAOS) members published **Guidance for utilizing Appropriate Use Criteria (AUC) in the management of the care of patients with orthopedic implants undergoing dental procedures** (JADA 2017; http://jada.ada.org/article/S0002-8177(16)30965-5/fulltext).

Appropriate Use Criteria (AUC) is a decision support tool to look at specific unique patient and dental procedure criteria and risks to determine the appropriateness of prophylactic antibiotic use. These AUC are for specific dental patients who have an increased risk of PJI, unrelated to the fact that they are undergoing dental procedure. (There are other AUC for other clinical orthopedic situations)

This **online only** decision support tool (bookmark it on your office computer) can be consulted at anytime. The Web location for the AUC for a dental patient with a prosthetic joint is: **https://aaos.webauthor.com/go/auc/terms.cfm?auc id=224995&actionxm=Terms** (accept the "terms" and you will be linked to a page to enter the needed patient and procedure specific information for the

PREVENTION OF ORTHOPAEDIC IMPLANT INFECTION IN PATIENTS UNDERGOING DENTAL PROCEDURE

dental appointment. The AUC algorithm will calculate if antibiotic prophylaxis is appropriate and advise on antibiotic choice if needed.

The authors note that AUC are not a standard of care and do not substitute for clinical judgment.

The patient and procedure specific criteria and risks requested by the algorithm are:

- Planned dental procedure's risk of bacteremia
- Immunocompromised status of the patient
- Level of glycemic control (related to diabetic patients)
- History of a periprosthetic or deep prosthetic joint infection (PJI) of the hip or knee that required an operation
- Time since the hip or knee joint replacement procedure was done

Prior to the creation of the AUC decision tree, dentists were advised to consult with the patient's orthopedic surgeon when making prophylactic antibiotic decisions. **Now it is appropriate for the dentist to make the final judgment to use antibiotic prophylaxis for patients potentially at higher risk of experiencing PJI (independent of dental treatment) using the AUC as a guide, without consulting the orthopedic surgeon.**

PREVENTION OF ORTHOPAEDIC IMPLANT INFECTION IN PATIENTS UNDERGOING DENTAL PROCEDURE

It should be restated, the clinical/evidence-based reasoning behind the current 2015 recommendations and the new 2017 AUC:

1. There is evidence that dental infections are not associated with prosthetic joint infections.

2. There is evidence that antibiotics provided before oral care do not prevent prosthetic joint implant infections.

3. There are potential harms of antibiotics including risks of anaphylaxis, antibiotic resistance, and infections like *Clostridioides* (formerly *Clostridium*) *difficile*.

4. The benefits of antibiotic prophylaxis may not exceed the harm for most patients.

5. The individual patient's circumstances and preferences should be considered when deciding whether to prescribe prophylactic antibiotics prior to dental procedures.

It should also be noted that, if the orthopedic surgeon recommends antibiotic prophylaxis or the patient prefers it, despite the dentist's recommendation against premedication, the prescription should be provided by their orthopedic surgeon or their physician, and they should take it under that clinician's direction.

PREVENTION OF ORTHOPAEDIC IMPLANT INFECTION IN PATIENTS UNDERGOING DENTAL PROCEDURE

Prophylactic Antibiotic Regimens (if the algorithm suggests that their use is appropriate):

Patient can take oral medication

If no allergy to penicillin:

Amoxicillin 2 g, 60 minutes before the dental procedure

If allergic to penicillin*:

Cephalexin** 2 g, 60 minutes before the dental procedure

  - *OR* -

Azithromycin 500 mg, 60 minutes before the dental procedure

See all **Notes** next page.

Patient cannot take oral medication

If no allergy to penicillin:

Ampicillin 2 g, IM or IV, 60 minutes before the dental procedure

  - *OR* -

Ceftriaxone 1 g, IM or IV, 60 minutes before the dental procedure

PREVENTION OF ORTHOPAEDIC IMPLANT INFECTION IN PATIENTS UNDERGOING DENTAL PROCEDURE

Patient cannot take oral medication

If allergic to penicillin*:

Ceftriaxone** 1 g, IM or IV, 60 minutes before the dental procedure

- *OR* -

Azithromycin 500 mg, IM or IV, 60 minutes before the dental procedure

*Note: Clindamycin is no longer the recommended alternative drug of choice for prophylaxis to prevent PJI, if the patient is allergic to penicillin.

**Cross reactivity of cephalosporin antibiotics in patients with penicillin allergy is 5% for first generation drugs and 1% for third generation drugs. These drugs should be used unless there is a history of anaphylaxis with penicillin administration. If there is a concern, patients should be referred for allergy testing prior to administering antibiotic prophylaxis.

It bears repeating, the ADA 2015 recommendations make it very clear that there is no scientific evidence documenting the value of prophylaxing any dental patient for the intention of preventing a prosthetic joint infection. The AUC is designed for people who have a high risk of PJI, **independent** of a dental procedure. The expert committee feels, in some dental situations, it is appropriate to prophylax such patients when they are having a dental procedure

REFERENCES:

American Dental Association guidance for utilizing appropriate use criteria in the management of the care of patients with orthopedic implants undergoing dental procedures. *J Am Dent Assoc.* 2017;148(2):57-59. Available at http://jada.ada.org/article/S0002-8177(16)30965-5/fulltext

Sollecito TP, Abt E, Lockhart PB, et al. The use of prophylactic antibiotics prior to dental procedures in patients with prosthetic joints: Evidence-based clinical practice guideline for dental practitioners-a report of the American Dental Association Council on Scientific Affairs. *J Am Dent Assoc.* 2015;146(1):11-16.

ANTIRESORPTIVE AGENT-INDUCED (BISPHOSPHONATE) OSTEONECROSIS OF THE JAW (ARONJ)

At this point in our knowledge of this disease, March 2018, there is not a lot of evidence-based information upon which to make clinical treatment decisions. All prevention/treatment information is based on expert opinion, which, by the way, though it is the best that can be gathered, is one of the lowest forms of scientific evidence. Below is "best guess" information, otherwise known as expert opinion, on prevention and management of ARONJ/BON. The below information comes from the current guidelines from the American Dental Association guidelines (2011) and the American Association of Oral and Maxillofacial Surgeons (2014).

KEEP READING THE SCIENTIFIC LITERATURE. RECOMMENDATIONS WILL MOST CERTAINLY CHANGE/BE REFINED AS EVIDENCE ACCUMULATES!

PREVENTION OF ARONJ/BON:

1. Patients should be in good oral health. Less oral problems seems to lead to less oral problems. See them before they start meds, clean up any problems, see them for the rest of their lives.

2. Drug holiday / Drug-free period. There is no strong evidence that a drug holiday is of benefit, but discontinuing the bisphosphonate for 3 to 6 months, if possible, is not inappropriate. Only the patient's physician can discontinue the drug.

3. Prophylactic antibiotics for surgical procedures. There is no documented concensus protocols as to antibiotic choice, dosage, or timing. Most agree good hygiene, starting antibiotic a day or so before the procedure, and continuing it for 3 to 5 days or until the mucosal surface has sealed the wound, is appropriate.

ANTIRESORPTIVE AGENT-INDUCED (BISPHOSPHONATE) OSTEONECROSIS OF THE JAW (ARONJ)

4. Chlorhexidine mouth rinse, 2 times per day until area is fully healed (4 to 6 weeks). Again, there is no evidence it helps, but "it is simple, inexpensive, and has no serious contraindications," is the way the experts phrase it.

5. Primary closure should hasten the creation of an oral mucosa seal. That would be good. But extension of the surgical site to accomplish primary closure expands the wound and may increase the risk of ARONJ/BON. That would be bad. So, primary closure, if simple and doesn't expand the wound.

6. Sharp bony margins should be conservatively rounded over to avoid mucosal trauma.

Note: The above suggestions are for prevention, <u>not</u> treatment or management of ONJ. If a patient gets ONJ, they should be referred to an oral surgeon (That is why they invented oral surgeons, for just such situations!) or a medical specialist with experience in managing such a disease. Please realize that the management of ONJ is very much a developing knowledge base, with no set protocols.

REFERENCES

Hellstein JW, Adler RA, Edwards B, et al. Managing the care of patients receiving antiresorptive therapy for prevention and treatment of osteoporosis: executive summary of recommendations from the American Dental Association Council on Scientific Affairs. *J Am Dent Assoc.* 2011;142(11):1243-1251.

Khan AA, Morrison A, Hanley DA, et al. Diagnosis and management of osteonecrosis of the jaw: a systematic review and international consensus. *J Bone Miner Res.* 2015;30(1):3-23.

Ruggiero SL, Dodson TB, Fantasia J, et al. American Association of Oral and Maxillofacial Surgeons position paper on medication-related osteonecrosis of the jaw--2014 update. *J Oral Maxillofac Surg.* 2014;72(10):1938-1956.

Wynn RL, Meiller TF, Crossley HL, eds. *Drug Information Handbook for Dentistry.* 25th ed. Hudson, OH: Wolters Kluwer Clinical Drug Information, Inc; 2019.

DENTAL DRUGS OF CHOICE FOR PREGNANT AND BREASTFEEDING PATIENTS

Risks from drugs to the fetus of a pregnant patient are twofold; first are teratogenic effects, which lead to birth defects. These risks are greatest during the first trimester when the child is being formed. The other risk is fetotoxicity which can occur any time during the pregnancy.

Risks from drugs relative to breastfeeding are primarily concerns of toxicity.

Below are key medication considerations from an excellent review article which provides greater detail: Donaldson M, Goodchild JH. Pregnancy, breastfeeding and drugs used in dentistry. *JADA*. 2012;143(8):858-871. Another excellent resource is an ADA Oral Health Topic review focused on Pregnancy: https://www.ada.org/en/member-center/oral-health-topics/pregnancy

Pregnancy and Breastfeeding "safe drugs"

Safe means safe to the fetus or baby, if the mother is taking that drug. All drugs have risks and, for example, clindamycin may cause problems for the mother, but is not a risk for the fetus or child, if the mother is taking the drug.

Analgesics

- Acetaminophen
- Oxycodone (avoid close to delivery and while nursing)

Antibiotics

- Amoxicillin
- Cephalosporins
- Clindamycin
- Metronidazole
- Penicillin

DENTAL DRUGS OF CHOICE FOR PREGNANT AND BREASTFEEDING PATIENTS

Local Anesthetic*

- Lidocaine (with or without epinephrine)
- Prilocaine

*Epinephirine dosages found in dental anesthetic cartridges are safe assuming it is not injected IV (larger amounts of epinephrine, used in some medical situations, are unsafe.)

Pregnancy "unsafe drugs"

For me it is easier to remember the unsafe drugs and just avoid them when treating pregnant patients. **Note:** The FDA Pregnancy Drug Category designations started to change to another system as of June 2015 and the old pregnancy risk category designations are no longer being assigned to new drugs. But the old system categories are still true and provide some guidance, especially for drugs used in dentistry, which have not changed a lot in years. (https://wikem.org/wiki/Drug_pregnancy_categories)

Analgesics

- Aspirin
- Glucocorticoids (prednisone)
- Ibuprofen (all other NSAIDs)

Antibiotics

- Doxycycline (tooth staining)
- Tetracycline (tooth staining)

DENTAL DRUGS OF CHOICE FOR PREGNANT AND BREASTFEEDING PATIENTS

Local Anesthetic

Articaine and mepivacaine must be used with caution. Bupivacaine and articaine are not considered compatible with breastfeeding.

Sedatives

- Benzodiazepines (ie, Valium, Xanax, Halcion, etc)

Breastfeeding "unsafe drugs"

Avoid: Aspirin, Doxycycline, Tetracycline, Benzodiazepines, and Diphenhydramine

Most drugs used in dentistry are safe when used with caution, relative to risk to the child, if the patient is breastfeeding. A good source of information is http://www.breastfeedingbasics.com/articles/drugs-and-breastfeeding.

9) TOBACCO CESSATION

Nicotine Replacement Therapy
Bupropion (Wellbutrin SR)
Varenicline (Chantix)

TOBACCO CESSATION

As a healthcare provider, you care. Tobacco use causes multiple health problems. You can help. You can intervene; take 3 minutes and ask the 5 "A's". If you get patient resistance, stop the discussion – do not push the patient past their comfort zone on this topic, it is counterproductive. Ask them about tobacco use the next time they come in, they may be more receptive.

1. **A**sk about your patient's tobacco use
2. **A**dvise to quit
3. **A**ssess for readiness to quit
4. **A**ssist if ready to quit (drugs, substitutes below)
5. **A**rrange for follow-up care (the patient should arrange for counseling - it helps a lot)

Nicotine Replacement Therapy (NRT) (eg, Nicorette gum, Nicoderm patches, inhalers, or lozenges) is available OTC and can be safely used to reduce cravings and withdrawal symptoms. It should be done in conjunction with counseling or some type of support, even self-counseling with available literature, to get the optimum outcome. NRT, alone, is less effective than the prescription drugs, but also has less adverse side effects.

Tobacco cessation is a complex psychological and physiological process. Though dentists and hygienists have a duty to the patient's overall health once they have done the 5 A's listed above, they may elect to refer the patient to a physician for pharmacologic intervention.

Tobacco Cessation Websites:

http://www.cdc.gov/tobacco/data_statistics/fact_sheets/cessation/quitting/index.htm
(comprehensive and informative resource from the Centers for Disease Control

TOBACCO CESSATION

Rx   **Bupropion** (Zyban [DSC]; Wellbutrin SR) **150 mg**

Disp   60 tablets

Sig   Starting 1 week from quit date, take 1 tablet per day for 3 days, then take 1 tablet 2 times per day (at least 8 hours apart) for 7 to 12 weeks (maximum dose: 300 mg/day)

> **CAUTION:** Read prescribing information. Many contraindications and warnings/precautions. Have patient review side effects on package insert (you should read them also). Instruct patient that if side effects occur, to stop medication and contact you.

– OR –

Rx   **Varenicline** (Chantix) **1 mg**

Disp   60 tablets

Sig   Starting 1 week before quit date, take 1/2 tablet per day for 3 days, then 1/2 tablet 2 times per day (at least 8 hours apart) for 4 days, then take 1 tablet 2 times per day (at least 8 hours apart) for 11 weeks

> **CAUTION:** Read prescribing information. Many contraindications and warnings/precautions. Have patient review side effects on package insert (you should read them also). Instruct patient that if side effects occur, to stop medication and contact you.

The #1 Dental Reference with over 500,000 Copies Sold!

The *Drug Information Handbook for Dentistry* is designed for dental professionals seeking information on commonly prescribed medications and dietary supplements. In this user-friendly resource, drug and natural product monographs are organized alphabetically and cross-referenced by page number. Dental-specific fields of information, such as Effects on Dental Treatment and Local Anesthetic/Vasoconstrictor Precautions, are highlighted in red, providing the ability to locate information quickly and efficiently.

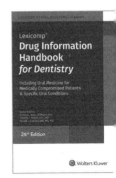

Editors:
Richard L. Wynn, BSPharm, PhD
Timothy F. Meiller, DDS, PhD
Harold L. Crossley, DDS, MS, PhD

ISBN: 978-1-59195-382-1
26th Edition
$99.95
Soft cover

Also available electronically for your mobile devices and desktop computer.

For more information or to place an order, call 1-855-633-0577 or visit https://store.wolterskluwercdi.com/

Lexicomp® Online for Dentistry
An Extensive Clinical Resource for Dental Professionals

Office-wide access to trusted Lexicomp drug information and drug interaction analysis.

- Searchable content from the #1 rated *Drug Information Handbook for Dentistry*, plus the entire Lexicomp dental reference library
- Daily content updates with the latest medication information
- Dental-specific drug interaction screening tool is designed to save time when checking for interactions and help reduce the risk of adverse drug events
- Lexicomp supports safe medication decision making when administering local anesthetics, antibiotics and analgesics

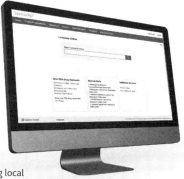

Access a Free 14-Day Trial of Lexicomp Online for Dentistry
No Obligation
(no charges or cancellation fees)
Call toll-free 1-855-633-0577, or visit
www.wolterskluwercdi.com/support/contact

For more Information or to place an order, call 1 855-633-0577
or visit https://store.wolterskluwercdi.com/

Lexicomp® Mobile Apps for Dentistry

Lexicomp mobile apps for dentistry provide instant access on mobile devices to point-of-care information. Advanced navigation tools make it easy to find clear, concise information when you need it most. Updates to our content are available on a daily basis, supporting your medication decision making with timely and clinically relevant information at your fingertips.

- Dental Lexi-Drugs includes information on over 8,000 medications, OTCs, and herbal products

- Up to 55 fields of information per monograph, including U.S. Brand Names and Generic Names, Special Alerts, Use, Local Anesthetic/Vasoconstrictor Precautions, Effects on Dental Treatment, Dental Dosing for Selected Drug Classifications, Drug Interactions, Dental Comments, and more

- Available complementary databases include Drug Interactions, Natural Products, and more.

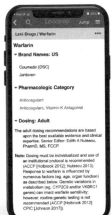

  Android

For more information or to place an order, call 1-855-633-0577 or visit https://store.wolterskluwercdi.com/

Lexicomp DENTISTRY OFFERINGS

At Wolters Kluwer, we understand that no two patients are alike, presenting individual challenges for optimizing treatment. These challenges require a wide range of resources that are clinically relevant and available at the point of care in a variety of formats.

Lexicomp dentistry knowledge areas include:

- Drug Information for Dentistry
- Drug Interactions
- Natural Therapeutics
- Dental Implants
- Clinical Dentistry
- Clinical Endodontics
- Clinical Periodontics
- Oral Soft Tissue Diseases
- Oral Hard Tissue Diseases
- Oral Surgery
- Pediatric Dentistry
- Office Medical Emergencies
- Patient Education
- Drug Identification

Our information is available in a variety of electronic formats and in our reference library of dental print titles.

For more information or to place an order, call 1-855-633-0577 or visit https://store.wolterskluwercdi.com/

I am delighted that you have found my little dental drug booklet useful (at least, I hope it was useful). And thank you for your help over the years. The booklet has grown based on your practical, practice-oriented suggestions.

If you have any edits, suggestions, or topics you would like added, please let me know at my email address, by snail-mail, or by phone. I will try to incorporate the information into next year's edition.

If you have a dental pharmacology/drug question or oral medicine/medically complex patient management question, please email me. This is a full service book and electronic application, complete with a live author. I am happy to research the question and respond.

Thank you.

Peter J.

Peter L. Jacobsen, PhD, DDS
Diplomate, American Board of Oral Medicine
Adjunct Professor, Dept. of Dental Practice and Community Service
University of the Pacific, Arthur A. Dugoni School of Dentistry
415-921-2448
415-921-0484 (fax)
pgjacobs@pacbell.net (best contact mode)
www.peterjacobsen.com (website)

NOTE!

The Little Dental Drug Booklet is *not* like **fine wine**.
It does *not* improve with age.

The LDDB is revised yearly to ensure you have the most up-to-date information in the ever-changing world of dental pharmacology.

Be sure you always have the latest edition!

Ordering information: Call 1-855-633-0577, visit https://store.wolterskluwercdi.com/CD or available at many App Stores